D0571476

PATIENTS WHO TROUBLE YOU

PATIENTS WHO TROUBLE YOU

WILLIAM A. STEIGER
M.D., F.A.C.P.
*John A. Kolmer Professor in Community
Medicine and Professor of Clinical Medicine,
Temple University School of Medicine*

A. VICTOR HANSEN, Jr.
M.D.
*Associate Professor of Psychiatry,
Temple University School of Medicine*

*Little, Brown and Company
Boston*

COPYRIGHT © 1964 BY WILLIAM A. STEIGER AND
A. VICTOR HANSEN, JR.

ALL RIGHTS RESERVED. NO PART OF THIS BOOK MAY BE REPRODUCED
IN ANY FORM WITHOUT WRITTEN PERMISSION FROM THE PUBLISHER.

LIBRARY OF CONGRESS CATALOG CARD NO. 64-22986

SECOND PRINTING

R 727.3
.S83
1964

INDIANA
UNIVERSITY
LIBRARY

NORTHWEST

Published in Great Britain
by J. & A. Churchill Ltd., London

PRINTED IN THE UNITED STATES OF AMERICA

PREFACE

This book is about people, people who are patients and people who are physicians. It is the result of many years of experience in treating patients and in teaching medical students, residents in medicine and psychiatry, and practicing physicians to understand their patients and themselves better. Because we have seen, time and time again, this increased understanding bringing better results for more patients with less strain on the physician, we decided to write a book about it. If *you* have difficult patients, incurable patients, disabled patients, or undiagnosable patients (and who does not?), this book is intended for you.

We fully recognize that there are many medical publications. There are books on diseases, on water balance, on metabolism, on neurosis, on the mechanisms of the unconscious, but only a few about people. There are innumerable medical case reports in which the only personal statement about the patient is that he is "well developed and well nourished." This book, in contrast, is about the people — the doctors and their patients — who are the underlying reality of *every* case report and of all medical books. They are presented in a disguised and condensed form, to be sure, but they are nonetheless real and alive.

How does one write a medical book about people? A book not about their electrolytes, or hormones, or Oedipus complexes — but about their character and personality? We struggled with this problem for quite a while, and began by writing down the rules and the laws for understanding character patterns and personality. However, we soon saw that this approach would give us just a book about rules and laws but not about people, so we dropped it.

We then decided to present a story — one of three physicians and their patients. One of these physicians, a young man just beginning, has much to learn about the private practice of medicine. The other two are mature, skilled men faced with the many problem patients of a busy, successful practice. Although the patients of all three are presented in brief sketches, the reader should be able to recognize them as the real people they are. Our story shows that these patients are often puzzling, frequently frustrating, and sometimes even infuriating to their doctors. We hope that our story also shows helpful and practical therapies for these troubling patients.

We have long been aware of the many heavy, technical tomes about medicine, psychiatry, and psychology. We have tried to write our book differently — with a minimum of technical jargon and even with some humor. We hope you will find what follows helpful, illuminating, and enjoyable.

We thank Francis H. Hoffman, M.D., for his frequent counsel, Mrs. Robert H. Nixon for editorial suggestions, and our wives for their encouragement and patience. We are especially indebted to Miss Cecelia Tluck and Miss Marie Walther for their perseverance with the many retypings of the manuscript, and to Mary L. Hansen, M.D., for her painstaking corrections of the manuscript and proofs.

W. A. S.
A. V. H.

Philadelphia

CONTENTS

Preface   *v*

Introduction to Chapters 1–3   *1*

1. PATIENTS, DOCTORS, AND PROBLEMS   *5*

2. MULTIPLE CHOICE   *13*

3. LEARNING BY DOING   *20*

Introduction to Chapters 4–12   *27*

4. THE IMPORTANCE OF UNDERSTANDING
    CHARACTER PATTERNS   *29*

ix

5. PEOPLE TEST 35

6. THE PATIENT WHO DOESN'T TRUST 38

7. HATE THAT PATIENT 42

8. THE SEDUCTIVE PATIENT 46

9. LIFE IS A PAIN 51

10. THE MARTYR 56

11. ANXIETY 62

12. SOMAPHOBIA 67

Introduction to Chapters 13–16 73

13. CUM GRANO SALIS 75

14. CONSCIENCE 79

15. WAY OF LIFE 83

16. DEPRESSION 88

Introduction to Chapters 17–21 93

17. WISHING WON'T MAKE IT SO 95

18. THE FAMILY 100

19. HUMPTY DUMPTY 104

20. YOU ARE NOT SICK 112

21. THE PROBLEM OF MEDICAL DISABILITY 115

Introduction to Chapters 22–24 123

22. THE CRYSTAL BALL 125

23. THE PLACE FOR PESSIMISM 129

24. NEVER UNDERESTIMATE THE POWER
OF . . . 132

25. THE UNCERTAIN DIAGNOSIS 135

26. DEATH, DYING, AND DIGNITY 140

27. INSTANT DIAGNOSIS 147

EPILOGUE 152

Introduction to Chapters 1–3

The young physician, finishing his education, has spent his working life in the world of the cognitive where knowing facts, solving problems, treating "cases," evaluating objectively, and taking examinations are the measures of the man. He has not realized that his prized cases, "worked up" so diligently on the wards, primarily as an intellectual exercise, are a highly selected sample of the total sick population that will course through his office. He knows little of the realities of hospital privileges, the rites of referral, the intricate economics of billing, of prepaid insurance plans, of income tax, of the organization of his office. Although he wants his patients to like him, he thinks that such a subjective basis for success is phony, unscientific. He eschews the bedside manner, preferring science to art, elaborate study to empathic understanding.

1

It is no wonder that many medical-school graduates who enter private practice, especially general practice, become frustrated and feel cheated. Raised in an atmosphere devoid of economic problems, family concerns, or financial demands, the realities of practice may seem unreal, even undignified to this "scientist." After all, in his long educational process, he has probably never made a house call, never dealt with a chronically ill patient for longer than a few months, never been continuously on call for his patients seven days and nights every week. Until now many of his patients did not know his name nor he theirs. He notified their families when they were about to die by writing "critical notice" on the chart order sheet. He argued and pleaded with, persuaded, and cajoled their families, whom like as not he had never seen before, for permission for an autopsy upon their dead member. The impersonality of his behavior never really occurred to him.

Moreover, the impersonality of modern society's view of man as an object had not been called to his attention, and, if it had been, he might well not have understood it. His frame of reference had always been Cartesian — man is an object in the world, to be weighed, measured, and analyzed as any other object. Man, the subject, with his private thoughts, feelings, anxieties, expectations, looking out at the world was almost unknown to him until he entered private practice.

In Chapters 1, 2, and 3, young Joseph D. Evans, M.D., begins to awaken to some of these ideas. He sees that the type of his practice — the kind of patients he sees — depends largely on the physician as a person and not solely on scientific knowledge, that all lacerations are not in reality handled alike but that the attitude of the lacerated person and its effect on the situation are significant. Finally he looks back to a medical-school experience when a psychiatrist made positive use of his own subjective feelings to define quickly the nature of his patient's problem.

Joe Evans is beginning to see that good medicine cannot be merely objective, that each patient is individual, and that the doctor-patient relationship is the interaction between two individual persons. Joe is finally comprehending the truth of what his religion taught him to believe, viz., that man is more than an object, he has a soul.

1. PATIENTS, DOCTORS, AND PROBLEMS

> JOSEPH D. EVANS, M.D.
> announces
> the opening of his office
> 407 East Elm Street, Preston
> For the general practice of medicine

WHEN DR. JOE EVANS finished his training at University, he and his wife, Sally, decided to settle in Preston. Having selected their house and done some remodeling for the office, they joyfully "hung out the shingle." The house with its office is at the beginning of "Doctors' Row," in the 400 block of Elm, east of Main, where it is quiet and shady. Although the house is old and gingerbready,

Sally and Joe think the high-ceilinged rooms and dark wood lend an air of professional dignity and stability.

One reason for Preston's appeal to Dr. Evans is its two good hospitals, the Memorial and the Community. Whereas Memorial boasts of a new and modern maternity wing with rooming in, it is not thought to have as high scientific standards as Community. Joe wisely got staff privileges at both.

Across from Joe and Sally's home is a house painted all white with some statuary in the front yard. At the front steps is a well-lit sign "S. Chernas, M.D." Dr. Chernas, Joe learned, is neat, even dapper, of medium height and every inch the professional man. He is positive in his manner, appears assured about his diagnosis, and is ready with a medicament for everything. He does all his work at the Memorial Hospital. His practice consists largely of hard-working people who man Preston's mills and factories. Medically they are unsophisticated with little understanding of the complexities of specialization and the process of referral. Dr. Chernas is their doctor; they expect him to handle any problem that comes along and for many years Dr. Chernas, assured and intrepid by today's standards, has done just that.

Early in Joe Evans' career in Preston, he was skeptical of Chernas' methods, although he had to admit to himself that he envied Chernas' large and faithful following. After a few years Joe changed his mind, finding Chernas a capable physician well suited to his clients, who did well by them within the imposed limitations of his practice. Joe further learned that Dr. Chernas had supported himself through school by working in Preston's mills thereby acquiring an understanding of his patients that could be gained in almost no other way.

On the corner below Joe's is a rambling three-story house with a high, well-manicured hedge. It has a side entrance which is decorated by a quiet, printed sign that reads: "M. Preston MacDonough, M.D." Dr. Mac-Donough, a descendant of the town's founder, is Chief of the Medical Staff at Community. He has a reputation of being very thorough. He generally does a meticulous history and physical examination and then orders several studies, which his office is well equipped to do, before committing himself to a diagnosis.

Although the younger set of Preston, who raise their children by Spock and Gesell and who like their Martinis with lemon peel instead of an olive, do not go to Dr. MacDonough often, to the ladies who sip a sherry, and their businessmen husbands who are always too busy at the office or the club, Dr. Mac-Donough is Sir William Osler. When he says "there is nothing organically wrong," they are better; if he says "this medicine will lower your blood pressure," the pressure falls. Whenever a doctor in town needs help, say, to persuade a patient to undergo surgery or to assure a family everything that can be done is being done for a sick member, Dr. MacDonough is the man to call in consultation.

When Joe had Dr. MacDonough see some of his hospitalized patients, he felt that he benefited from MacDonough's experience and authority. Then one day, seeing one of these patients, an elderly lady, going in to Mac's office, Joe was upset. That night, to his surprise, she was in his office. When Joe asked about the visit to Dr. MacDonough, she was embarrassed and hastened to explain that it wasn't that she did not like Dr. Joe or that he wasn't a good doctor, but that Dr. MacDonough was older and so, she thought she would go to him. Dr. Mac, praising Joe highly, had refused to see her, however, and insisted she return to Dr. Evans.

Joe will never forget his first house call, shortly after he had opened his office. It was about 11 P.M. when Dr. Chernas called and asked him if he would go over to Sherman Street near the river to see a patient. Joe went in a hurry, and Sally said she'd wait up. He had a bit of trouble finding the house and wondered why the devil people didn't ever have numbers one could see. When he knocked on the door, a man in his undershirt answered. Joe said, "I'm Dr. Evans. Dr. Chernas asked me to come," and got the reply, "She's upstairs."

Joe found his patient, fortyish and fat, occupying most of the bed in a dimly lit front bedroom. She had a little fever and a dry cough, but after Joe gave her the most thorough examination she probably ever had, he could find nothing else. His mind raced with ideas — tuberculosis, atypical pneumonia, fever of unknown origin? He wished he could get an immediate white blood count and a chest x-ray, as he would have at University. Finally the patient said, "All the kids have this, too, Doc. I guess it's a 24-hour virus." Relieved, Joe agreed with her diagnosis and prescribed aspirin and elixir terpin hydrate.

When Joe went downstairs, he reassured the patient's husband that his wife had only a virus infection. Her husband wasn't impressed and said gruffly, "That's what I told her it was. Should I pay you now?" This caught Joe off-guard and he found himself embarrassed. "Oh," he said, "I'll send you a bill." When he got home, Sally told him he should have taken the money.

Joe did some insurance exams, made occasional house calls for Dr. Chernas, talked with all the detail men, and treated a salesman for gonorrhea (who didn't want to go to someone who knew him) . Then, happily, his chance came to show off his University training, or so he thought. His patient, a spinster in her fifties, had had abdominal pain for several years and had seen

all the doctors in town — even M. Preston Mac-
Donough — without getting help. Joe first thought of
porphyria, a rare hereditary metabolic disorder, but
the patient's urine-screening test was negative for
porphobilinogen. (He wished the more complex and
specific spectroscopic exam for porphyrins done at University was available at Memorial or Community.) He
ordered upper gastrointestinal x-rays, and these, too,
were negative. While puzzling over the diagnosis, he
received a call from the patient. She was obviously
angry. She said, "I have spent all that money for the
tests and I'm no better. As a matter of fact, I am worse,
and I think the x-rays burned my stomach lining.
When are you going to do something for me that will
get me better — or are you just like all the rest of
the doctors, no good?" Joe was flustered and embarrassed. Nothing like this had happened to him before.
He tried to explain that there was nothing wrong with
her, but she would not listen, said she'd go to someone
who wasn't a greenhorn and really find out what was
the matter. That ended that. Joe always wondered,
though, whether the spectroscopic analysis of her uri-
nary porphyrins would have shown ————.

This patient was not the last Joe saw who did not
seem to fit into any textbook description. He saw those
that were tired all the time, those who threatened to
go across the street if he didn't give them penicillin,

the "lady" who called him to her apartment late at night for no good medical reason, the ones who would not do what he said they should, the healthy who persisted in being sick and disabled despite his best efforts, and so on. Even M. P. MacDonough, with his beautifully equipped office, went to bed occasionally puzzled over some of the patients he had studied carefully in whom he could find no organic disease. Was there something he was missing? And Dr. Chernas found time from his busy practice to ask Joe Evans some casual questions about what they thought at University.

DR. C.: What is abdominal migraine like?

Dr. E.: Professor ——— didn't believe in it.

DR. C.: Had a patient who was tired, listless, anorexic for six months; thought it was functional, but could infectious mononucleosis last that long?

DR. E.: Would look for brucellosis.

DR. C.: Brucella agglutination test negative.

DR. E.: Oh!

At first, as Joe's practice grew, he sometimes wished that he had stayed at University with all its interesting cases. Why weren't all his cases mitral stenosis, lymphoma, lupus erythematosus? Was he missing them? He didn't think so. It was just that many of his patients were different from the selected ward cases. Their problems were often different, too. Not only that, but as he got busier, those night calls became rather wearing after a full day, and he found himself looking for someone younger to help him. When these young men, out of respect for his knowledge and gratitude for his help, called him in consultation, he found that some of their patients tried to come to him, the older man, as they once did to M. P. MacDonough.

2. MULTIPLE CHOICE

HERE ARE THREE QUESTIONS with multiple-choice answers that Joe Evans never encountered in a medical-school test, licensing examination or specialty board certification:

A. The fifteen-year-old daughter of the Chief of the Medical Service suffers a one-inch laceration of the forehead. The wound is most likely to be sutured by:
1. The intern in the Accident Dispensary
2. The surgical resident
3. The Chief of the Surgical Service.

B. A chronic alcoholic falls while inebriated and sustains a one-inch laceration of the forehead. The suturing will likely be done by:
1. The intern in the Accident Dispensary

2. The surgical resident
3. The Chief of the Surgical Service.

C. A patient complains of ill-defined, poorly local-
ized abdominal distress. A gastrointestinal x-ray would
most likely be ordered if the patient is:
1. Someone on public assistance, seen in the teaching clinic of a University Hospital
2. A handyman with five children and no medical
   insurance
3. An elderly lady in a nursing home
4. A busy physician.

These questions illustrate that, as Joe Evans soon
learned, the practice of medicine is not so simple, so
precise, so "scientific" as a standard textbook might
portray. It is complicated by social, vocational, economic, and emotional factors. These areas have been
called *the art of medicine*. It has been largely assumed
that the *art* cannot be taught, except by example, and
cannot be learned, except through experience. It is
one of the purposes of this book to demonstrate that
the so-called art of medicine can be approached scien-
tifically and that it is both teachable and learnable.

The following formula describes the "chemistry"
that goes on between the doctor and his patients:

$$Patient + Doctor \rightleftarrows Plan\ of\ management$$

The major portion of this book deals with the first term of this formula, the patient. It discusses some different types of people who are patients and the problems they constitute for the doctor. It outlines examples of appropriate plans of management for these different people. Since the success or failure, the acceptance or rejection, of this management vitally affects the doctor-patient relationship, the formula is written as a reversible reaction.

What of the doctor in the following equation? For one thing as he gets older and more experienced, he tends to become a constant. Then the formula can be written for him:

$$\text{Patient} + \text{Constant} \rightleftharpoons \text{Plan of management}$$

This constancy can be either limiting or useful. Thus the internist may use almost exclusively wet soaks and penicillin to treat a furuncle, whereas the surgeon tends largely to incise and drain. This is an instance in which special training can reduce flexibility. Or because of personal bias the physician who cannot stand neurotic women will largely eliminate them from his practice — or by our formula:

$$(\text{Neurotic women}) + (\text{Doctor who cannot tolerate them}) \rightarrow (\text{Discourage them from coming back})$$

According to this formula, which of the following reactions is more likely to go to successful completion?

(Immigrant laborer) $+$ (Dr. MacDonough) $\rightleftarrows$
$\qquad\qquad$ (Successful plan of management)

or

(Immigrant laborer) $+$ (Dr. Chernas) $\rightleftarrows$
$\qquad\qquad$ (Successful plan of management)

Student physician Adams, the only child of a husband-wife team of research scientists, thrived in the intellectual atmosphere of his home. He was a member of Phi Beta Kappa and had been president of the debating society of his small college, a school that prided itself on not having a football team. Adams did not dance and hardly dated, although he was a good-looking boy and proper in his behavior. His record during the first two years in medical school was brilliant. During his junior year, one of his first patients was a young, curvaceous sweater-girl with a vague pain in the left side of her chest. Adams insisted that her pain must be intercostal neuralgia, although it had no neuralgic characteristics. He seemed flustered when this fact was pointed out. Somehow, he had omitted examination of his young patient's breasts, although he usually was very thorough.

Adams needs to become aware of the anxiety aroused in him by the presence of an attractive young girl. Such awareness will help prevent his anxiety from interfering with his examination, diagnosis, and management. In fact, he can learn that the presence of such feelings is often the direct result of the personality of his patient (cf. Chap. 8).

Dr. Sarnik's parents were poor but industrious. He worked his way through school by playing in a jazz band at night, working on a construction gang in the summer, and selling his Rh-negative blood. He was a good, conscientious physician but he had one blind spot — he could not tolerate patients who were seeking compensation for illnesses or accidents. "Getting something for nothing, that's the whole trouble with our country," he always said in his lecture to them. His wife could tell when he came home at night that he had seen such a patient that day and she was careful not to cross him. His colleagues, too, told him to take it easy. "You can't fight City Hall!" But to him such patients always remained a personal affront.

It would be wise if Dr. Sarnik and others would ask themselves "Why do I feel the way I do about this patient? Is this my problem, my way of reacting to all such people? Or is it this patient's problem?" Most important, "I will not allow these feelings of which I am aware to interfere with my objective handling of this patient's problem."

These examples illustrate that each physician is a product of his personality and his training. His reaction to a particular patient is a compound of his objective appraisal of the medical problem and his subjective reaction to the patient as a person. As the physician gains experience, his own subjective reactions become relatively constant. He can analyze his feelings toward his "patient-person," using them as a diagnostic and therapeutic tool — just as he develops his ear for murmurs or his touch for liver edges.

She was a little old lady with nondescript complaints who told in detail how her son and daughter-in-law mistreated her. Outwardly she deserved sympathy but somehow Joe Evans was annoyed by her. Irritated, he felt like giving her phenobarbital and hurrying her out of his office. He checked this impulse and treated her with care and respect. Later Joe met her son, who thanked him for his kindness to his mother and said he knew how difficult, demanding, and disgruntled his mother really was. Joe Evans' *feelings* of annoyance and irritation about the old lady were correct. He learned that he was a "constant" in the doctor-patient interaction. He could trust his *feelings,* as he trusted his physical findings, and be equally as objective about them, making sure that his feelings did not interfere with the proper management. Gradually Joe discovered that this awareness of his own feelings about patients increased his diagnostic acumen, broadened his therapeutic range, and saved him from the useless expenditure of energy.

Finally, everyone will agree to another expression of the same formula, viz.:

(Increased understanding of patient)+
(Increased knowledge of self) → (Better patient care)

The aim of succeeding chapters is to force this reaction to the right.

3. LEARNING BY DOING

WHEN JOE WAS A SENIOR at University, he had been called on to present a case to the staff of the Functional Clinic. He had not been happy with his assignment to this clinic in the first place. While his classmates were hearing murmurs in the Heart Clinic, reading x-rays in Radiology, and lowering blood sugars in the Diabetic Clinic, he was doing histories and physical exams on patients with no organic diseases. Nevertheless, Joe was picked to present a case. His patient's chief complaint was vague, lower abdominal pain. Joe had explored the pain in detail: its nature, timing, and relationship to meals, special foods, and bowel movements, without positive correlation. He narrated these in the History of Present Illness during the conference. The Systemic Review was also negative. Social History disclosed that his patient was a secretary who neither smoked nor drank. Family History disclosed no hereditary disorder. Joe told of the negative physical examination in which he described his patient as a "well-developed, well-nourished white female, looking her stated age of twenty-eight years and in no acute distress." Her laboratory and x-ray studies were normal, and a consultant from the Gastric Clinic suggested a "psychophysiologic gastrointestinal disorder." Since the consultant's prescription of a sedative-antispasmodic mixture and a bland diet brought no real relief, the patient had been referred to the Functional Clinic.

During Joe's detailed presentation, the instructor in psychiatry listened patiently. When Joe finished, he asked him, "What is she like?" Joe was taken aback by the question. He thought he had just finished describing the patient in great detail. The one thing further he could think of saying was that for a clinic patient, she was above average in intelligence.

The psychiatrist then asked Joe what he had done for her? Joe said that he had reassured her that she had no organic disease. He had explained to her that her examination and x-rays were negative, that she had no ulcer, no cancer, and so on. But the symptom persisted, and Joe was disappointed and even angry. This was evident when next he testily demanded of the psychiatric instructor, "What more *can* you do for her?" The instructor replied, "Let's go have a little talk with her."

PSYCHIATRIST (*to patient after opening pleasantries*):
Do you mind if I smoke?

PATIENT: No, not at all.

PSYCHIATRIST: Would you care for one?

PATIENT: No, thank you. I don't smoke.

PSYCHIATRIST: Oh?

PATIENT: My father would never permit it.

PSYCHIATRIST: He was pretty strict?

PATIENT: Well, he was, or is, a minister, you know. He never allowed smoking or dancing or things like that.

PSYCHIATRIST: Hmm.

PATIENT: I didn't really mind it, and after I left home and came to the city to work, I set my own standards.

PSYCHIATRIST: I wonder if this could be related to your trouble?

PATIENT: How's that?

PSYCHIATRIST: I wonder if you've been doing something or things recently that maybe you are not so proud of or that bother your conscience?

PATIENT (*a bit startled*): Do you think that this may be the trouble?

PSYCHIATRIST: Well, what do you think?

PATIENT (*obviously has something on the tip of her tongue but is hesitating to say it. With a rush*): I have been going with a young man, a teacher, we're engaged, unofficially, that is, and we've been doing, er, going too far. We've fought against it. He's really a fine person. We even decided one time not to see each other, but it didn't work. I worry about it all the time. I know it's wrong and if anything should happen, my father . . .

When Joe and the instructor returned to the conference, they related what had happened. The instructor explained that children of ministers are apt to acquire strict consciences which may bother them when they try to loosen the fetters. The knowledge that this patient was such a person permitted him to get to the area of trouble quickly. Moreover he had surmised from Joe's presentation that this patient was not the usual clinic patient, and when he saw her he felt a sense of social equality. This had impelled him to offer her the cigarette, something he was unlikely to do with the usual clinic patient. Then he wondered if this girl had come to the clinic because she was ashamed to go to a private physician; the clinic was more impersonal. These thoughts, feelings, and intuitions led to an interview that was quickly productive.

The instructor then turned his attention to Joe.

How much had Joe been reassuring himself when he presumably was reassuring his patient? Was he reassuring himself that he had not missed an organic disease? When the patient did not improve, it raised doubts in Joe's mind and consequently he got angry at her. But without a positive definition of her problem, what improvement could he expect? When a patient has pain, should telling her that it is not organic necessarily make it better? Finally, Joe's instructor pointed out how little understanding Joe had had of his patient as opposed to a group of organ systems. Joe's pride was a bit wounded by this experience.

Joe had other difficult experiences from which he learned a great deal. For example, shortly after he began to practice, a young married couple visited his office. They were both diabetic and were taking insulin. They wanted to know if they should have children. Joe, always proud of his knowledge and his scholastic ability, answered their questions in detail. He related the bleak statistics that forecast the likelihood of their children being diabetic and pointed out the high mortality rate in infants of diabetic mothers. His learned dissertation was suddenly interrupted by the loud sobbing of the young woman. Too late Joe learned that she was already three months pregnant.

Some time later, Joe saw a shrewd young man whose hypertension he was treating with Reserpine. When it became necessary for the patient to have a hernia repaired, he asked, "Should I stop my Reserpine before the operation?" Joe was about to answer that it wasn't necessary, when he remembered his previous painful lesson. Instead, he replied, "Why do you ask?" Thereupon the patient showed him a magazine article relating the hypotensive difficulties under anesthesia of patients taking Reserpine. Joe was glad he had answered the patient's question with a question.

The answering of patients' questions and giving advice was more complicated than Joe had anticipated. Sometimes the way a patient asked for advice was so flattering that Joe found the temptation hard to resist. At other times his sympathy would overcome his good sense. This happened when he forcefully urged an elderly widower, lonely and depressed, for whom he felt sorry, to move in with his daughter and son-in-law. Only later did he learn that the son-in-law was a difficult, argumentative, possibly psychotic person with whom his patient never got along.

Joe had a young patient who was somewhat unhappy in her marriage to an older man. She told this to a consulting gynecologist, who found her very attractive and who sympathized strongly with her feelings of marital dissatisfaction. He said to Joe, "Why should she stick to that old fogy? She's a darn good-looking, young woman." When Joe explained that this was his patient's second marriage, that she had previously divorced a man her own age, and that her present husband was a fine person, the consultant was amazed. Whether he realized that his own feelings of attraction toward the patient had dictated his impetuous advice, Joe rather doubted.

Joe learned again the importance of keeping personal feelings, preferences, and prejudices out of medical situations. Before he reassured a patient, he learned to ask himself: "Whom am I reassuring, the patient or myself?" Before he answered a question, he thought of what might be behind it. Before he gave advice about personal matters, he sought out all details of the situation; by then the patient was usually able to decide for himself.

Introduction to Chapters 4–12

The application of the methods of the physical sciences to man, the object, has resulted in many significant advances, especially in understanding him as a physico-chemical machine and in the conquest of disease. It has also, to man's detriment, influenced those dealing with behavior to spend their major energies in a never-ending search for an abstract universal, a basic principle, a simple causal determinant, an $E = mc^2$ that will explain all behavior. The history of man reveals that such efforts have always existed and that determinants are always found but that their truth has never been objectively confirmed or denied. Abnormal behavior has been attributed to spells cast by enemies, to the devil, to the gods, to the unconscious, to parents, and even to the psychological trauma of being born. This dealing in abstract concepts can be another way of avoiding the person of the patient and his realistic *problems. It is sometimes easier to think about egos, ids, superegos, past life history, and so on than to deal with current behavior and realistic present-day problems.*

We hope that in the succeeding chapters, the word pictures, or sketches of some common character patterns will foster the reader's recognition of these life styles and make him aware of his possible reactions to them. We are not concerned with the why *of the life style but are concerned with* what to do *when the patient's character pattern interferes with his function in society or with his proper medical management. We do not pretend to have a single, clear-cut, A, B, C, D approach to every one of these problems — there isn't any. In addition, the character pattern of the individual physician is as important as that of the patient in the decision of what to do and how to do it.*

4. THE IMPORTANCE
OF UNDERSTANDING
CHARACTER PATTERNS

JOE EVANS, observing his own work and that of other clinicians, concluded that the ability of a physician to diagnose and treat patients depends on the consistency of disease patterns and the predictability of their response to appropriate therapy. To illustrate: A patient complains of upper abdominal pain two hours after meals, severe enough to awaken him at 3:00 A.M., but relieved by the ingestion of alkali. This pattern of symptoms, their location, timing, and relief is consistent enough from patient to patient for the physician to predict, with a high degree of accuracy, that the patient has a peptic ulcer. Based on this pre-

dictability, the physician orders an upper gastrointestinal x-ray, not an intravenous pyelogram or an
electrocardiogram, and puts the patient on an ulcer
regimen. The yield from both the x-ray examination
and the diet is bound to be high because of the consistency of the clinical pattern of a peptic ulcer.

In like manner, Joe found that since the patterns of
people's underlying characters are consistent throughout life, their behavior can often be understood and
predicted. It is of special significance to physicians to
know that patients will handle their health problems
and react to illness much as they behave in other life
situations. Illness and deformity seldom change the
established personality or character pattern of an
adult, as will be seen by the following cases.

A disgruntled, very shy young man left home,
moved to a large city, rented a room, and found a
clerical position. He had made no close friends, joined
no groups, and dated no girls in the ensuing three
years. He then suffered a serious leg accident, resulting
in a surgical amputation below the knee. Despite a
good stump and a well-fitted artificial limb, he was not
successfully rehabilitated. He now had an obvious,
external reason to be shy and distant and to find it
difficult to work with other people.

Some who did not know this young man might say
that his amputation made him shy, that it was the

reason for his disability and his lack of social adjustment. His pattern of behavior before the accident, however, reveals that the amputation not only aggravated a consistent, life-long pattern of unacceptable behavior but justified its continuation.

Another example was Mrs. H. D., a woman in her fifties who called and asked Joe's nurse for an appointment. When the nurse inquired about the nature of her problem, Mrs. H. D. said it was none of her business, that she would tell it only to the doctor. She insisted, moreover, that she wanted a time when she would not have to sit waiting with a lot of other patients. When she saw Dr. Evans she told tearfully of the wonderful, contented life she had with her lovely house, her husband and children, until six months ago, when she had her hysterectomy, "that awful operation." She wondered if the surgeon had "botched the job," because since then everything has been impossible. She was always cranky and depressed and felt that she was no longer a woman. She did not take care of herself and let her appearance slide badly. When Joe sat back to listen and lit a cigarette, she asked him not to smoke; it had always disagreed with her.

Superficially, it would seem that this woman's life was delightful and gay until her operation. Actually, Mrs. H. D.'s intimate acquaintances knew, as Joe Evans knew when he listened to the clues and attended to his feeling of dislike for her, that she had always been disgruntled and unhappy. She had nagged her husband endlessly when he took an occasional night out with "the boys"; she was critical and severe with her children. Her husband had suffered with her problem of dyspareunia. In reality the operation did not change her personality. Instead it gave her the license to justify and increase her complaints.

If Dr. Evans accepts as absolute Mrs. H. D.'s statement that her operation (or the amputation in the previous case) caused her symptoms and her disability, he is faced with a very poor prognosis. The uterus (or the leg) cannot be put back. Such acceptance would be an inaccurate appraisal of the real situation and, furthermore, one behind which the patient can hide, so that the real personality problems are never faced. In both these cases, the biological problem was the match that kindled the conflagration; the tinder of the character patterns was already there.

The following two cases further illustrated to Joe how different character patterns can greatly influence the treatment, prognosis, and recovery of two individuals with the same medical diagnosis.

H. T., a retired bookkeeper, sixty-eight years old, suffered a typical coronary occlusion after shoveling snow. His four-week stay in the hospital was uneventful. He returned home asymptomatic and resumed his normal pattern of life.

V. W., a fifty-year-old man, had a coronary occlusion at the same time as H. T. During his hospitalization he was a problem — refusing to stay in bed, complaining of the food, and criticizing the nursing. After six weeks he was discharged to his home, where he has remained a semi-invalid.

Both men had coronary occlusions. Their cardiac evaluations, electrocardiograms, and rises in serum transaminase were fundamentally the same; their management, degree of recovery, rehabilitation, and prognosis were completely different. These differences resulted because two different people were involved. The disease was the same in each, but the character patterns of the patients differed markedly.

Mild-mannered H. T. had worked 40 years at the same routine job. He accepted his modest role in life and enjoyed its security. Any standard textbook details the treatment of his biological disorder which in his case was all the physician needed to know. By contrast, aggressive, competitive V. W. had risen to the position of vice-president in a small corporation by dint of an all-absorbing, lifelong effort. Never particularly liked, he was more feared than respected. Shortly before his heart attack a younger man had been promoted to a position higher than his, a position he believed he deserved. Although he never would admit it, even to himself, V. W. could only regard his being bypassed as evidence of personal failure. To return to work under such conditions was inconceivable. Consequently, he devoted almost full time to awareness of his heartbeat, the care of his bowels, and the taking of a great many nitroglycerin tablets. Whereas the management of his heart disease was relatively easy, the rehabilitation of his person was complex and difficult for it depended not on the condition of his heart but on his readiness to accept his job situation realistically.

Some questioning of V. W. or his wife about his thoughts on what brought on his heart attack might have revealed the source of his discontent. After he had got his anger "off his chest," his physician might side with him, "I don't blame you for being disappointed and angry. I wonder, though, if it isn't time you gave up some of the heavy burdens, especially now with your heart attack, and let a younger man carry some of the load?" Such a face-saving approach might permit V. W. to diminish his disability and resume a reasonable amount of activity.

Joe was daily seeing the importance of understanding the character patterns of his patients. His observations on some of these follow.

5. PEOPLE TEST

WHILE COVERING ANESTHESIA one night at Community Hospital, Joe Evans fell to chatting with Miss Gall, the seemingly ageless night supervisor on obstetrics. Complaining that Doctor Bombast was sending in a patient for delivery, she asked if Joe had ever noticed that the patients in obstetrics were like their physicians? Dr. Bombast was loud and crass, sometimes swore, even threw instruments when the situation was difficult. His patients were much the same, wailing loudly and complaining often. Although bitter exchanges sometimes occurred between doctor and patient, they blew over quickly. Despite the seeming chaos in the delivery room, Dr. Bombast's record as an obstetrician was excellent. Miss Gall compared him with Dr. Suave, the epitome of dignity and good breeding, who seldom raised his voice. During his deliveries there was rarely any commotion. His patients were generally "cut from the same bolt of cloth." Joe realized that a patient of one of these physicians would likely be uncomfortable as a patient of the other. He saw that much can be learned about a doctor from observing the type of patients he sees and, what is more important, that in answering a consultation, much can be anticipated about the patient by the personality of the physician who referred him.

There were many instances when Joe's assessment of a problem took into account the person who was relating it. For example, his own competent and loyal nurse-receptionist was invariably taken in by a hard-luck story; her protégés tended to be masochists, usually in an irretrievable mess. He encountered a different problem with the night nurse on 2 Main who personally conducted a one-nurse crusade against narcotics and hypnotics. Joe had to write specifically timed orders for these drugs because her idea of the amount of discomfort a patient should endure and his were miles apart.

Joe chuckled over one incident for some time. A high-strung intern, who foresaw the possibility of impending disaster in almost every situation, was called to see an emotionally upset, postoperative patient. What he did or said to the patient Joe never knew, but he did order Equanil. The patient became even more upset, claiming that the medication was making her worse. Unaware of the intern's visit, the surgical resident, composed and sure of himself, saw the patient, spoke calmly to her for a few minutes, and ordered Miltown. Thereafter, she quieted down and spoke of the marvels of the last pill she was given.

Joe called his observations of people his "People Test." It was often more help to him than laboratory studies and x-rays. After he had mastered the art of observing his patients and colleagues more objectively, he applied the same principles to himself. When he found an area to which he was particularly blind or especially sensitive, he took it consciously into account in order to improve his objective judgment.

6. THE PATIENT WHO DOESN'T TRUST

JUDY SAT ALONE in her room, mulling over her unhappy life. Damn those doctors and their restrictions; no cokes with the crowd after school,
no swimming in deep water. What did they know
about diabetes? She had it and they didn't — and she'd
had it for 10 years. She could regulate herself. Dr.
MacDonough was no different from the rest; she had
an appointment with him tomorrow and she knew the
routine — another lecture on following that lousy
diet. At this point Judy ate a candy bar, her second that
day. Oh well, she'd say she felt "shocky" from a too-low
blood sugar. Later she would take some extra insulin
to cover it.

Judy resented her doctors, thinking that their every

recommendation was devised to torture her. Her doctors, who sometimes responded in kind, got especially angry because they were frequently called to treat Judy for diabetic coma or hypoglycemic shock. Why in heaven's name didn't she take care of herself and save them the repeated anxiety of possibly losing her?

Next day, Dr. MacDonough was almost relieved when Judy did not keep her appointment and spared him the need to scold her again. Nevertheless he was worried about her. What would become of her? Should he have been less stern? Under her tough, rebellious exterior was she really a frightened kid who felt she couldn't rely on anyone? He decided that he had better have his nurse get her on the phone.

Over the years, Joe learned that not every patient trusts physicians. Some went to more than one doctor at the same time. They would ask Joe's opinion about the other's medicine and he knew that they checked on his advice in like manner. Some didn't like him to write down their confidences. A few patients reacted in a bizarre, subjective manner to almost any medicine prescribed — as if it were poison.

Joe Evans had a patient who was an engineer, precise and mathematical. He often stayed late at the office, checking and rechecking the work of his subordinates. He treated Joe Evans the same way, demanding minute explanations of everything Joe did to him and for him. He was wary of medicines and said that even aspirin constipated him. When a nurse gave him an unexpected injection one night in the hospital, he was alarmed, feeling certain that it was a mistake. The following morning he complained that he felt miserable all over. Joe finally said, "You don't seem to have faith in me. You are always questioning all the details of my treatment." The patient *said* that he did trust the doctor but that, in his business, he had to watch every detail. If he or his subordinates made a mistake, a bridge would fall down — "but, ha, ha, the doctors are lucky, they bury their mistakes." Joe told him firmly that the way he ran his business was up to him, but that his treatment was his doctor's business. This discussion, plus a *reasonable* amount of explanation, and occasional reassurance for his doubts, resulted in satisfactory cooperation.

A fifty-two-year-old man had Paget's disease of the skull since he was twenty. He was typically deaf and, as a result of the bony overgrowth, had a huge head, which, since no ordinary hat would fit, he covered with a cap, adding to his grotesque appearance. He had stopped working and spent most of his time at home. He had sought help from numerous physicians over the years but none could stop his skull from growing. His faith in people, including his physicians, was at a low ebb. He now believed that even aspirin and vitamins

made him weak, "affected his system." Joe asked this
man to trust him, said he understood how difficult,
embarrassing, and even frightening his condition must
be — but the patient never returned after the second
visit. He probably had felt that he should try the new,
young physician in town, but did not return when he
learned that Joe had no new magic for his problem.

Joe Evans found that if he paid attention to the *kind
of* person who came into his office *and to his own feelings about them* he could sense (rather quickly) the
wariness of those who did not trust him. He could
almost feel their need to maintain a psychological dis-
tance. If this attitude did not interfere with their
management, no special measures were required.
When proper medical management was endangered,
however, he would quickly discuss their lack of faith.
Judy might have benefited from such a talk with Dr.
MacDonough. Certainly it helped Joe in treating the
engineer's cardiac condition. Joe didn't become angry
with patients who didn't completely trust him because
he knew it was their temperament and not a personal
reaction to him. Calm discussion and not angry re-
crimination or rejection was in order.

7. HATE THAT PATIENT

JACK ABRAMSON had been Joe Evans' classmate at University where Joe knew him to be a good medical student, conscientious, interested in his patient. One day Jack had come out of the clinic examining room in a rage. With flushed face, he told how hostile and insulting his patient had been. First, she had asked him, "Are you an intern or a doctor? — You look just like a boy — how can you possibly understand my problems? — I don't like to be practiced on." The instructor told Jack of similar experiences as a student, of his wounded pride, and how little these things meant in retrospect. Jack calmed down a bit and when the instructor assured him that he was a good doctor, pointing out that the patient ridiculed him even before she had known him, he had to smile. Her behavior was not really personal; she would have done it to any student. When Jack returned to the examining room he said, matter-of-factly, "Well, I hope you got it all off your chest — now can we get down to your problem?" Disarmed by his refusal to fight, the patient replied, "I don't know why I acted that way" and her management went satisfactorily thereafter.

Nick was a tough, hard-nosed truck driver who gave everyone on the ward and in the clinic of Memorial Hospital a difficult time. He would not shave and he rarely bathed. He frightened the nurses, threatening to knock them across the bed if they hurt him when giving an injection. The resident staff disliked him, called him uncooperative, swore that he enjoyed ill health, and groaned when he came on the ward. At times, Nick demanded that only the Chief treat him and if he didn't, Nick would not take his medicine.

Nick had severe, rapidly progessive hypertension that hadn't responded to medication or a Peet sympathectomy — Nick never let the staff forget this. At times he would threaten to go to another hospital, to which someone would reply, "Well, why don't you?" Nick was hostile to the staff and the staff was hostile in return. One resident would not allow him in the ward; another said that he was too busy to be bothered.

Several times a week Nick heard the doctors on rounds say that the antihypertensive measures had failed. He was edematous now, as well as hypertensive.

He heard and saw how diet, oral diuretics, mercurial diuretics, cation exchange resins, aminophylline, hypertonic glucose, and so on failed to rid him of the edema. Finally Dr. Chernas came on as Chief of the Ward Service. When he heard about Nick's actions, he really laid him out. He told him that if he was going to act like a gorilla, he would be treated like a gorilla. What did he think this was, a flophouse?

Nick got the idea. He began to shave, to smile, to help the nurses on the ward. Everybody was happier; Nick was easier to manage even though he was still very sick. When one of the nurses asked Dr. Chernas how he handled Nick so successfully, Chernas said, "Hell, that big bluff is scared to death. I knew him in the mill. He always was a bag of wind."

Different physicians handle angry patients according to their own talents. Dr. MacDonough generally draws his long white coat about him and becomes haughty with them. Dr. Chernas uses the direct approach, saying "What the hell is the matter with you? Let's cut this stuff out and stick to business." With Chernas' patients, who are familiar with such language, this approach works well; with Dr. MacDonough's patients, it would be offensive.

Dr. Evans, as he gained experience and became self-assured, was able to sit back and listen to the angry patient without getting upset. When a patient saw that he was not being threatened and that he was being understood, medical management was generally better. Joe realized that in the past the anger aroused in him by some patients had interfered with proper, scientific management. Now when he got angry with a patient, he made sure that his recommendations and treatment were based on rational medicine and not on emotional reaction.

8. THE SEDUCTIVE
PATIENT

J OE EVANS remembered well the experience of two of his classmates with a very attractive patient, the talk of the class. She was a twenty-eight-year-old divorcée with a captivating smile and fine figure who visited the University Comprehensive Medicine Clinic and was given prompt attention for her headaches. She had a blood pressure of 220/140. As a hospital bed was not available, she was treated as an outpatient. With medication and diet, her blood pressure fell to 160/100 and her headaches disappeared. While being investigated for specific causes of hypertension (i.e., renal disease, pheochromocytoma, etc.) she recounted her sexual experiences to the two medical students, disclosing that she had been married to a sadist who assaulted her constantly and that she had also been intimate with a number of men, including her sister's husband.

She fascinated the students and they spent hours with her. To them she was misunderstood, the victim of a cruel life, and they were overzealous in helping her. Their interest and enthusiasm were not on a scientific basis of responding to the patient's need, but a result of her seductive manner.

In his practice, Joe never had a patient who tried to be sexually seductive, but he was aware of being seduced in a number of other ways. For instance, a thirty-five-year-old, unmarried woman with diffuse abdominal pain, had had six operations for this and related complaints, mainly gynecolgic procedures, resulting in the removal of her uterus and ovaries (cf. The Martyr, Chapter 10). During the course of her visits she brought Joe a present that he knew she could ill afford. She told Joe of sexual involvement with several men who would not consider marrying her. Joe pointed out to her the repetitive, self-defeating pattern of her life. In reality she had a very low opinion of herself and so great was her need for acceptance, that she would offer her body, and, in his case, a gift. After this talk and several others she could see quite clearly how unsuccessful her pattern of life had been and altered it considerably. Joe never did find the cause of her abdominal pains, but after a while they disappeared.

It is the custom of many patients to give gifts to their physicians, especially during the holiday season. The acceptance of an occasional small gift is generally harmless. Some presents, however, are obviously uncalled for and, as a matter of fact, a discussion of these gifts may be necessary in order to handle the case. The following is a case in point:

An elderly widow was the family matriarch. She kept her children under her thumb in a quiet but effective way by bestowing gifts and money, providing vacations, paying for help during sickness, and so on. In return she demanded obeisance and a great deal of attention. On occasion, when her family did something that displeased her, she would get upset and make it clear to all about her that the misdeed was worsening her heart condition. As she had marked cardiac disease, the device was most effective.

When Joe pointed out this pattern to her, she denied it vehemently and was sick in bed for two days afterward. On his next visit she presented him with a gift for his wife. This, of course, was again an attempt to control the situation as she had so often done with her family. Joe asked if their previous discussion had upset her. She was able to admit that she had seriously thought of disengaging him from the case, but instead had decided to get him a present.

Seduction by flattery was tried by a new patient,

referred for a consultation, who opened the interview with Joe by stating that the doctor certainly had an excellent reputation, especially for one so young, must be very brilliant, and that he was *sure* that the doctor would find out what was wrong and fix him up.

A widow, fifty-one years old, was successfully treated for a hematologic disorder. She always thanked her physicians profusely for what they did and repeatedly implied that they were next to God. Periodically, however, this seemingly adoring patient would insist that her blood be examined, although there was no clinical evidence of recurrence. When asked why she was still concerned, she admitted that she suspected her blood disease was venereal in origin. When she was assured that this was not so, she still insisted on a blood test. Some time later she developed a cancerphobia. X-rays and examinations disclosed no abnormality but she insisted that her doctors were so nice, so kind, they wouldn't tell her if she did have cancer. When shown the x-ray report, she wondered if the doctor had had a false report typed up just to reassure her. (Cf. The Patient Who Doesn't Trust, Chapter 6).

Patients who call their doctor God can be just as unrealistically negative if they do not get their way as they are unrealistically positive. These positive feelings, on the part of the physician as well as the patient, can be as much of a deterrent to good management as can hostile feelings. The physician's feelings should not be allowed to interfere with his central control processes. His head, not his heart, should determine what is to be done for the patient.

9. LIFE IS A PAIN

AMANDA LOWERED HERSELF heavily into the chair at University Clinic. She glanced briefly at the student doctor in his starched white coat and grunted. (He had studied her thick chart for some time and was still puzzled as to just what was wrong. Most entries listed a complaint or two and then a prescription. Rarely was there a specific diagnosis. What disease did she have? What would he treat? Her blood pressure was up sometimes, so maybe he could prescribe Reserpine. She was obviously obese and needed a diet. That would help the osteoarthritis in her knees, too.)

STUDENT DOCTOR: What is your chief complaint, Mrs. Jefferson?
PATIENT: Huh?

STUDENT DOCTOR: Er, what's bothering you? What's
your trouble?

PATIENT: Them other doctors say I got high blood.

STUDENT DOCTOR: Anything else?

PATIENT: Well, I got arthritis, I think.

STUDENT DOCTOR (*getting irritated*): Do you hurt
any place?

PATIENT: Uh, huh.

STUDENT DOCTOR: Well — where?

PATIENT: Where?

STUDENT DOCTOR (*giving up*): You better get undressed so I can examine you.

PATIENT: I have to get undressed?

This somewhat caricatured conversation is familiar
to every student and practicing physician who has
worked in a metropolitan clinic. Everyone tries hard
initially to find some specific disease to treat. When the
patient is seen in the Medical Clinic, she usually ends
up after many studies getting phenobarbital. She often
has high blood pressure but seldom do the intravenous
pyelograms, the Regitine tests, and so on disclose a
remedial abnormality. Moreover, the blood pressure
seems to stay about the same over many years despite
blandishment with every new antihypertensive agent,
singly or in combination.

In the Gynecology Clinic her lower abdominal pains

are chronic inflammatory disease of the pelvis. In the Orthopedic Clinic her low-back pain defies all the belts and braces. In the Diabetic Clinic she swears that she sticks to the prescribed diet, but she never loses weight. In each clinic, and she attends several, she is studied and studied — but the studies do not seem to get her cured. She makes up a large proportion of those patients known as "crocks." She arouses anger and frustration in the students and staff, who gladly refer her to other clinics or dump her on Social Service at the slightest opportunity. When Joe Evans finished his training at University, he felt that he would never see such crocks again and he was glad. Only later did he realize that private practice has its share, but here they pay their way.

She was a little old lady of Russian birth who always got off on the wrong foot with her doctors. First she enumerated all the big-name "professors" who had treated her in her younger days and then she moaned through a myriad of complaints. No sooner had one symptom been remedied than another sprang up. The doctors felt her name-dropping was derogatory and they were frustrated by her chronicity. "If she isn't satisfied with me, let her go to see the professors she's always talking about," was their attitude.

Norma Jean had a pretty name but little else to go with it. She had thick lips, a thick body, and heavy legs.

Her feet hurt her all the time, even though she encased them in orthopedic oxfords. In rapid-fire fashion she told of her complaints, always vague and difficult to pin down. Consequently her doctors always felt uncertain and were afraid they might be missing something organic. This resulted in numerous studies and consultations that ruled out a multitude of diseases but resulted in no certain positive diagnosis.

The doctor's dilemma with these patients is in taking their complaints too literally. If he feels that every complaint must have a medical diagnosis, he leads his patient through a maze of diagnostic channels and usually ends up where he started. Only now, without a precise diagnosis, he is impotent to help the patient and resents him for it. In actuality these patients are bemoaning their lot in life; they are bellyaching about their misery.

Amanda was one of twelve children of sharecropper parents. She had helped in the fields from the time she was five until she escaped by marriage. She had worked all her life, scrubbing floors, cleaning up other people's dirt. Her husband, often without work, had become increasingly shiftless. She barely managed to eke out a living for her family, had no savings and few possessions. She was old beyond her years, "pooped out," and ready to retire.

Our little old lady, too, had come upon hard times

since her husband died. When she bragged about her previous physicians, she was not attempting to demean her present physicians but rather was begging them to recognize her as a person of substance. The red-carpet treatment and a few words of sympathetic understanding were the indicated therapy.

Norma Jean's symptoms were her calling card. They got her into the clinic. She liked to tell the doctors about all the sacrifices she had made staying single, caring for her aged parents and her sick brother. These people were now dead and she needed someone to tell her that she had been a good girl, to reassure her periodically, and to urge her to carry on.

Patients like Amanda may have medical problems and deserve careful medical evaluation, but one can be sure that often their complaints are social and should be so recognized without undue delay. The appreciation that some patients express their difficulties in life in medical symptoms can save a lot of wear and tear on the doctor and the laboratory.

10. THE MARTYR

S HE DOESN'T HAVE MUCH MONEY," explained the gynecologist, "but she needs help." Dr. Mac-Donough said, of course, he would see her, do what he could and keep his fee to a minimum.

She was middle-aged, plump, and dowdy, had high blood pressure, and was nervous. Below her short-sleeved housedress, her elbows were covered with scaly red patches. When Dr. MacDonough commented, "I see you have psoriasis," she sighed. "Oh, I've had it for years and tried a lot of things, but nothing cures it, so I don't do anything about it anymore." She took care of her high blood pressure in the same way. When asked about her nervousness, she said, "I have a problem — my husband drinks. Why, I don't know. I do everything for him. Every night he either goes out to a taproom or sits in front of the TV and drinks beer."

All this was said in a whining voice. Although Dr. Mac-
Donough felt sorry for her, he was still annoyed. He
was wondering why in Heaven's name she put up with
her husband's indifference and abuse, when she volun-
teered, "I only do it for the children's sake, and sometimes I'm not even sure they appreciate all I've gone
through for them. I'm worried right now that he'll be
coming home drunk. I never know — and every day I
worry how he'll be when he gets home. I wouldn't be
here this afternoon if the woman specialist hadn't insisted. I don't think anyone can help me, doctor, and I
hate to take pills. If I get a headache I just suffer it out,
I don't even take aspirin." MacDonough, at this
point, felt his own pressure rising. What could he do
with this woman who did so little to relieve her suffering? She didn't take pills, wouldn't take aspirin, stuck
with her drunken husband — wait until he saw that
gynecologist! MacDonough was not too disappointed
when she failed to show up for her next appointment.

A sixty-three-year-old woman complained to Joe
Evans of lack of appetite, difficulty getting to sleep,
and fatigue, especially in the morning. His initial impression that she was depressed was augmented by
finding out she had some ideas of self-destruction and
dreamed of dead relatives. His examination disclosed
only a nontoxic symmetrical goiter; blood count,
blood sugar, cholesterol, urinalysis, chest x-ray, and

basal metabolic rate were normal. The patient had been an extremely hard worker all her life. She had worked every day with her husband in their restaurant, rising at 4:30 A.M., as well as keeping house and raising three fine children. She was especially proud of her outstanding record as a blood donor during World War II. Two years before she came to see Dr. Evans her husband sold their business. Her husband took a job from 8:00 A.M. to 5:00 P.M. while she stayed at home. Meanwhile her children had married and had moved into their own homes — her place in the sun was gone. She felt worthless; no one needed her. She became depressed. Her children saw it and loyally rallied around. They took their mother out for rides; they did everything they could for her and told her to take it easy. "Why should you spend all day Sunday in the kitchen cooking for the whole family? We'll take you out for dinner, Mom."

Dr. Evans' plan of management was to reassure the patient about her health and explain that her sickness was one of spirit. He praised her for her many wonderful contributions in the past and told her that she needed to continue them. He instructed her family to give her some responsibilities, such as baby sitting. These discussions led to her taking an active role in the charity affairs of her church where her business acumen was useful. At first, she had to push herself, but as she became more active, her depression lifted. One year later she continued to be well and was active in a number of charitable groups. Obviously this woman had a great many assets. She had always been a working, contributing individual. Once her problem was pointed out to her, Dr. Evans could expect that she would achieve health just as she had achieved her other goals in life.

A sixty-one-year-old woman complained of having almost every body ailment. Her examination, blood count, urinalysis, blood sugar, and chest x-rays were negative but when Joe questioned her about her home situation she poured out her anger and dissatisfaction. She had been a slave at home, always cooking, cleaning, washing and never getting out, unappreciated — her twenty-four-year-old unmarried son couldn't do anything for himself, she still did her married daughter's laundry, and so forth. On one visit she complained of a severe headache. It developed after baby-sitting for her daughter, when she got "burned up" at her daughter and son-in-law for going out and "blowing-in" twenty-five dollars in one night. It turned out that, while baby-sitting, she could not refrain from scrubbing the kitchen floor and washing the dirty dishes, all the time muttering about her daughter's sloppy housekeeping.

Joe knew that this type of patient could get the doctor angry. He might be tempted to berate her for her slavishness or to shout at her, "What do you want to do — kill yourself?" Actually this reponse does nothing except punish her — and she is already doing a good job of that on her own. The physician should not get trapped into punishing such a patient; instead, he should do as Dr. Evans did, let her make the choice. He told her that she can go on "doing" for everybody, if she wants, or she can begin saying "no" to baby-sitting, children's laundry, etc., and "do for herself." She must make up her own mind. The conflict is hers, but getting sick is no way to resolve it. Getting sick will not get her the appreciation she seeks; it will only irritate people.

Managing the Martyr

1. Do not make a martyr out of a martyr. If you get angry at him, attack him, threaten him, or deride him, you place yourself in the same position as everyone else in his life.

2. Be particularly conservative about performing surgery on these patients. Martyrdom is the character pattern of so-called surgical addicts.

3. The mother who has devoted herself entirely to her children, who has sacrificed all other interests for them, will often become depressed when they leave home. This is the time to channel her energies into other activities (such as nurses aide, women's club, church, or bridge).

4. The martyr who is married to an alcoholic or a sadist is difficult to change. Suggest either learning to live with the situation or leaving it, but point out that sickness is no way out.

5. To the martyr there is no satisfactory solution. If she continues to do everything for everyone, she carries an impossible burden; if she stops she is lost, since she knows no other way of relating to people. This dilemma should be discussed openly with her.

11. ANXIETY

MRS. THERESA CULLEN was wracked with anxieties and to Dr. Evans she poured forth a long list of fears, which she dated back to the birth of her second child. She had thoughts that she might harm her baby — drop her or get poison in the formula. She refused to go into the kitchen because of the knives, could not look at TV or read the papers because of the violence in them, could not stay alone and had to call her husband home from work increasingly. She was certain that she was losing her mind.

Several physicians had reassured Mrs. Cullen it was only nerves, but they and their tranquilizers had proved of little help. After several panicky calls to them in the middle of the night, they had made it fairly plain that they preferred not to be bothered any longer and that she should get hold of herself, advice that served only to increase her anxiety.

By the time she came to Dr. Evans, the patient, her husband, and her family were desperate. Initially Joe was annoyed at his nurse for squeezing her in between previous appointments, but as he listened to Mrs. Cullen's story and recognized the severity of her anxiety, he understood the haste. First he pointed out the obvious — that she was terrified; that the entire situation was snowballing downhill; that it was time to stop and, without panic, to take stock of the situation. He pointed out firmly that although she may think so, in reality she was not losing her mind. Despite her fears of the worst, no disaster had occurred. Perhaps her past experiences could prove to her that although her anxieties were most uncomfortable, *nothing* had really happened; the things that she feared, harm to the baby and death for herself, had not really occurred. He pointed out that, although her fears were irrational and not based on fact, she would continue to have attacks of anxiety for some time because there was no magical formula for their immediate cessation. He tried next to get her to see the difference between thought and deed — because she had bad thoughts about her baby did not mean that she had to act on them or that she was a terrible mother. He finally asked her to promise him that she would do nothing rash or foolish, a promise she gave with some trepidation.

Although Dr. Evans seriously considered placing Mrs. Cullen in a mental hospital, he thought it could be done at a later date if necessary. Encouraging her to try to make a go of it seemed the more optimistic approach. He discussed the decision fully and openly with the patient and her husband and they agreed to try it and also to have her see Dr. Evans once a week. To reassure her further of his support, he gave her his telephone number with permission to call him anytime she wanted. If he was busy at that particular minute, he promised to call back as soon as he could. Meanwhile she was not permitted to call her husband at work; if she felt that she just had to call someone, she should call Dr. Evans.

This regimen helped diminish Mrs. Cullen's fears. Although things were shaky at first, she gradually gained confidence in herself through experience. Dr. Evans was initially apprehensive about permitting unlimited phone calls, knowing the troubles with calls her other physicians had had. Oddly enough, the reassurance that she could call was usually enough to forestall her calling at all. In the months that followed, she called once at 2:00 A.M., possibly to test his sincerity. When he responded pleasantly, she apparently needed to call no more at night, nor did she abuse the privilege during the day.

Anxiety, which brought this patient to Joe Evans, is one of the most common motivating forces bringing patients to physicians, yet conversely it is often the force that keeps patients away. Unless the physician recognizes this paradox and handles it properly, he may inadvertently make it difficult for a patient to get adequate medical help.

A sixty-year-old foreign-born woman came to the Gynecology Clinic at Memorial Hosiptal one day with a large external prolapse of the uterus. Obviously, she must have been aware of this condition for a number of years. The resident physician, unaware of her fear of both her illness and its consequent treatment, saw only the abnormality and immediately urged an operation. The poor soul became so terrified that she fled the clinic never to return. Joe Evans wondered if the outcome would have been different had the resident appreciated how frightened the patient was of hospitals and surgery. Handling her irrational fears should have been the first step in preparing her for surgery.

A seventeen-year-old unmarried girl sought medical attention in the second trimester of her pregnancy, during which she had gained considerable weight. The physician who saw her was alarmed at her obesity and spoke to her sharply about it. When she gained another five pounds, he threatened her with the horrors of hell and described the toxemia of pregnancy. (The possible serious consequences of her condition had made him anxious and he became angry at her as a result.) Terrified, she now put on even more weight so that on her last visit the obstetrician threatened to refuse treatment unless she cooperated. At this point he pulled out all the stops in his misguided, although sincere, effort to gain her cooperation. Shortly thereafter her anxiety became so overwhelming that a psychosis resulted.

We have seen that anxiety in the patient can bring him to the physician or can prevent him from seeking medical care. Recognition of and dealing with this anxiety are often necessary before further medical steps can be taken. Anxiety in the physician can, in like manner, motivate him to work harder for his patient or can diminish his scientific skillfulness.

12. SOMAPHOBIA

JOHN WORTHINGTON had always been considered an odd person. From a wealthy family and educated at the best schools, he apparently did well as a respected but somewhat distant bachelor until the age of thirty-eight, but for the past eleven years, he has neither worked nor associated with people in the community. Instead he has concentrated his attention chiefly on his heart and on going from doctor to doctor. At present, Mr. Worthington is an authority on the current cardiac literature and sometimes appears, at least on the surface, to have read more than his doctors.

In his frequent visits to physicians, he has never returned to one who told him that "there was nothing wrong" with him. Whenever it was suggested that he return to work, John would counter with "Can you guarantee that I don't have myocardial damage and won't get a heart attack?" Any physician who would admit even a bare possibility of heart damage would become the fair-haired boy for a short period of time, because John felt that he could then continue his social isolation with the excuse of "doctor's orders."

John Worthington lives in constant dread that he is going to have a heart attack and die. In reality, his disability is not his cardiac condition, whatever it may be, but his fear. It is fear that disables him, that needs recognition and treatment. Although John has had no objective evidence of heart disease, his situation would not change if he had. Fear — not some cardiac disorder — would still be the deterrent to his rehabilitation.

Martha Kane was a thorn in the flesh of all the physicians whose help she endlessly sought. An intense young woman, she was always convinced that she was suffering from some serious disease. When Joe Evans heard that Martha had married, he dreaded the possibility of her becoming pregnant, foreseeing his own involvement in her care. In due time she conceived and bore a son after a hectic pregnancy.

Shortly thereafter she brought the infant to Joe for a checkup with a long list of fears and complaints — the baby wasn't eating enough, wasn't gaining properly, was becoming ill, and it was her fault. Joe wondered if raising the baby was too much for her and asked if the baby should be put up for adoption. As he had expected, she declared vehemently that she would never consider such a possibility. Joe then pointed out that when confronted with the logical outcome of her own words, she made an emphatic decision to the contrary. For the first time Martha saw the futility and absurdity of her usual reaction to stress, and with Joe's help was able to make some important changes in her behavior. She learned not to become disturbed over every minor difficulty. Joe, in return, spent some extra hours patiently teaching her how to care for her child.

Some of the most difficult patients to help are those with somatic obsessions, the result of anxiety, and the list of medical problems in which anxiety is the basic problem is long. For example, the teen-ager who fears to socialize presumably because of acne; the young matron who is extremely fearful of getting pregnant; the young matron who is so fearful she won't get pregnant that her marriage is in a turmoil; the colitis patient who is afraid to go out lest he be caught without a bathroom, and so forth. These fearful, pessimistic people, who always find something to worry about, see disaster ever looming. Their world is a frightening one. The fear of socializing, of getting or not getting pregnant, of going out is a manifestation of their fear-

fulness. It is fear that needs treatment. Sole attention
to the acne, to the glands, or to the colitis will rarely
remedy the disability.

In managing these patients whose anxiety is the
major cause of disability:

1. Don't tell them that nothing is wrong — something is. They are literally scared to death. It is helpful
to point out that they are incapacitated more by fear
than by actual physical impairment. "The only thing
we have to fear is fear itself."

2. They often go from doctor to doctor and tend to
accept that doctor who gives the most serious and
pessimistic medical diagnosis, which confirms their
fears and permits them to continue their present pattern. Unfortunately, they follow the advice that increases their disability — staying home and resting,
not going back to work, and so on.

3. Advice should be explicit; the vague "Take it
easy" can be crippling.

4. It may help to predict the dismal future that lies
in certain store if they continue in their current way
of thinking, if they continue to let fear disable them.
Their fear may confine them progressively to home,

to first floor, to room, to bed. The answer is not going to be another medicine or a new test or another medical opinion. The answer lies in how they handle their anxiety. It can either disable them or it can spur them on. They do have a choice.

Introduction to Chapters 13–16

Most religions have similar goals for mankind and yet throughout the centuries their disciples have fought with one another. They seem to forget their great similarities in fundamental concepts while magnifying their differences in form. Psychological systems and schools of psychotherapy appear to have much in common with religious sects. It is not our purpose to enter these disputations but rather to point out that, for the average physician, doctrinaire adherence to one system or one technique of psychotherapy is to be guarded against.

The succeeding chapters show that a technique which works for one physician may not be suitable for another. Dr. Chernas could never be a passive, reflecting mirror for prolonged periods. He is a man of action, but when he points his finger, berates or scolds, his underlying sincerity and warmth shine through. Dr. MacDonough, on the other hand, is too formal, too prim, to deal at length with the intimate emotions of others, and it should not be expected of him. Each of these physicians has devised his own method of dealing with certain problems and for each it is the most effective.

The next chapter illustrates Dr. Evans' process of arrival at his personal technique.

13. CUM GRANO SALIS

EVER SINCE HIS DAYS IN MEDICAL SCHOOL Joe had been troubled by the different psychiatric schools of thought. His school had been entirely psychoanalytically oriented, and after his initial period of revulsion, he felt that he could make some sense out of the Oedipus complex, childhood sexuality, and the like. However, his early attempts at applying these theories met with rather disastrous results. He recalled, particularly, two patients he had seen in the outpatient clinics.

The first was Arthur, a thirty-seven-year-old man, who had been in prison three times, once for armed robbery and twice for dope addiction. He was out of prison when Joe saw him, but not working, living with his wife and her mother. The family existed on a bimonthly public welfare check that was sent to his

mother-in-law. Joe reasoned that one of Arthur's difficulties was that he was not functioning in a masculine
role — he was living off the bounty and under the
thumb of his mother-in-law. His dependent role was
antithetical to being a masculine, aggressive male.
Arthur needed to be made a man. With much work,
many telephone calls, and more persistence Joe managed to have the public welfare check turned over to
Arthur so that he could budget the money, learn how
to be responsible — in short, be a man. The theory
seemed good to Joe, but any corner bartender could
have predicted the disastrous results.

The second was Annie, a regular at the University
Clinic for years. She was a chronic paranoid schizophrenic who came periodically because of her multiple
complaints. Everyone in the clinic knew Annie, toler-
ated her complaints, and handled her as expeditiously
as possible. After reviewing the chart Joe concluded
that her problem was loneliness and lack of love. He
decided he was going to give her the missing ingredi-
ent. Fired with enthusiasm he entered the waiting
room, flashed his toothiest smile, and gave her an ef-
fusive welcome. Poor Annie jumped up from the
bench, ran across the waiting room, screaming "Get
away from me; I know what you're after; get away from
me. . . ."

Shortly thereafter Joe went to the State Hospital for

six weeks' senior clerkship. Here the atmosphere was entirely different from the University. The majority of the staff were overtly against psychoanalysis and Joe saw many patients on electroconvulsive therapy and drugs, which were fundamentally scorned at his University. He was surprised how many of the acute patients improved by these means during the short time he was there.

When he entered private practice Joe was forced to take some kind of a stand. At first he vacillated between the psychoanalytic approach and the organic, sometimes combining the two. As time went by he concluded that he was not going to be able to settle the differences in the various schools of thought, nor did he have the experience or the background to evaluate them. He conceded that the various techniques might be useful in the hands of an expert. After all, reading a book on surgery and listening to some lectures do not qualify one to do a bowel resection. Perhaps psychiatry is the same. What he needed was a psychiatric first-aid philosophy that was practical for him with his patients.

During his busy office hours, he could not spend an hour with patients, but he did find that he could set some time aside for those patients who especially needed psychotherapeutic help. Then he had to get over the notion that listening and talking are not really doing anything, in order that he could charge adequately for his time. He soon found that most patients were grateful for his time and willing to pay for it. Many of his patients were helped by these sessions, so that Joe began to look forward to his psychiatric afternoon. He used drugs where indicated but recognized that his calmness, assurance, acceptance, and interest were the most potent therapeutic agents.

14. CONSCIENCE

IN MEDICAL SCHOOL Joe Evans had heard much about Freud and his theories, particularly his discovery of the ill effects of the repression of basic, biological drives. Once in practice, however, he got the impression that many people in Preston repressed their drives too little. There was, for example, the successful attorney, with a wife and three children, who came to Joe because of severe attacks of anxiety. He was having an affair with a younger woman and was considering leaving his family for her. Joe reassured him about his physical health and prescribed sedatives and tranquilizers liberally but with little benefit. Finally he referred him to a psychiatrist, who attempted to find out why this man was acting and feeling as he was. He analyzed his early childhood and his repetitive dreams, but after half a dozen sessions with no improvement the patient refused to return. Joe met this patient again a year later and found him much improved. When asked to what he attributed his betterment, the patient said that he had finally realized that he must live up to his obligations at home. He had given up the other woman, was spending more time at home and with his children, and withal felt a great deal better. The psychiatrist had suggested that he might have to make such a choice in order to get well, but he couldn't bring himself to a decision at that time and even resented the idea that getting better was up to him.

In retrospect Joe realized that he should have sized up the situation promptly and pointed out to the patient that he had always been an upright and moral person. He suspected that as long as he continued living a double life, his conscience would bother him and he would have symptoms. If he wanted to be well, he would either have to mend his ways or get rid of his conscience. It appeared to Joe that it was not repressed drives that made his patient anxious but an unsuccessfully repressed conscience.

Then there was a young man who had divorced his wife and was leading a gay life as a bachelor. He complained to Dr. Chernas of impotence, especially when bedded with the wife of a good friend. Chernas felt that it served him right and bluntly told him so.

A widow brought her teen-age daughter to Dr.
Chernas fearing that she might be pregnant. She told
about her daughter's disobedience, her late hours, her
fast friends, etc. The girl sat down in Dr. Chernas'
office, took out a cigarette and was about to light it
when Dr. Chernas entered. He immediately ordered
her not to smoke in his presence and told her to stand
up when an older person entered the room. Then he
berated her for her actions, for not obeying her
mother, told her graphically of the trouble she was
headed for, ordered her to go to church regularly and
live up to its tenets. Fortunately she was not pregnant and after Dr. Chernas' boost to her conscience,
her behavior improved.

Dr. Evans was not the type to brandish the warning
forefinger at such a patient as the girl just described.
He would see the girl on several occasions, would
suspect that her actions were motivated, at least in
part, by some negative feelings toward her mother,
and attempt to bring them out. He would have
pointed out that she was cutting off her own nose
(masochistically acting-out) and would have discussed
how to avoid disagreements with her mother. He
would have suggested that together they examine her
long-range goals in life and how she planned to at-
tain them.

Dr. MacDonough would probably examine such a

girl and then suggest that the problem was not a medical one, by his definition, and suggest that her mother take her to a priest or minister for counseling.

Any one of these techniques can be effective and the one used depends, to a considerable degree, on the personality of the physician. To recall our formula:

$$(\text{Patient}) + (\text{Doctor}) \longrightarrow (\text{Plan of management})$$

There are many people visiting physicians with symptoms consequent to their not living up to their own moral obligations, whether it be cheating on their income tax, questionable business deals, or taking unfair advantage of others. After all the erudite talk about conflicts, it may seem awfully simple to suggest that the trouble is a common conflict — a guilty conscience. Nevertheless, Joe and others found that if such a patient will follow the dictates of his conscience, he often will feel better.

15. WAY OF LIFE

MYRON LIEBER was forty-eight, a small man with bright, dark eyes and a quick mind, especially with figures. He made his livelihood, a good one, in "points." Joe learned that a point meant a percentage and as he got to know Myron he found that a few points here and a few there were the secret of much financial success.

Myron's complaints were not new. He had had "stomach trouble" for years, consisting of ill-defined epigastric distress and periodic diminution in appetite. His frequent insomnia was handled well with a sleeping pill. A recent decrease in libido had made him wonder if he were "changing life." His major problem, and he knew it, was chronic anxiety.

Myron asked Joe for a checkup, including an upper gastrointestinal x-ray. Several done previously had been negative, but Myron wanted to be assured that he had no ulcer or cancer. Joe, recognizing that his patient was a worrier, did as requested and when no abnormalities were discovered, Myron felt somewhat better. He had long since tried all the stomach remedies and tranquilizers and had settled for those he felt best for him — Joe only needed to approve of them. At that point Joe did not know what more he could do for the patient, but Myron asked if he could come in every two weeks and talk. Joe agreed and set the time aside. They discussed Myron's background, his problems in business, his family. Joe learned that Myron had seen a psychiatrist regularly for two years, and felt that the talks helped him although his symptoms were still present. As Joe listened, he found that Myron spent much time talking about his childhood. He had had a domineering, chronically ill father and possessive, demanding mother. He recognized his ambivalence to his parents, including his death wishes for his mother, his fear of authority-figures, which arose from his relationship with his father, and his feelings of insecurity consequent to the insecurity and poverty of his childhood. Myron had learned his psychiatric lessons well.

Joe was sympathetic toward Myron's past difficulties but believed that he was setting himself up as the

hopeless victim of a past he could not change. Joe
began to seek for Myron's current problems and
this is when he learned about points. Myron's life was
one of deals — he was continually involved in quick,
often risky, business transactions that held promise
of a fast profit. On one hand he had his wife and
children to whom he owed security; on the other,
he had the demands of his business for capital invest-
ment. Moreover, he always had interest to pay on
loans, fellow-investors to repay, options that were
running out, tax investigations, legal fees, political
payoffs, etc. Joe suspected, too, that sometimes new
money intended for project B was used to pay off demanding investors in project A.

Joe painted this synoptic picture of Myron's way of
life to him one day and said that he didn't wonder
that it made Myron anxious, knotted his stomach,
and left him with little libido at the end of the day.
Joe wondered what would happen if Myron had a
nine-to-five job and an assured paycheck? Myron replied, "Doc, if I were in the Army, I'd feel a hundred
per cent."

Myron, of course, did not change his way of life
and still has many anxious periods. He sees Joe
Evans periodically for checkups and reassurance and
they joke about Myron, the wheeler-dealer of Preston.

(Joe has been tempted at times to invest some money with him, but he fears that he might lose his objectivity — and his money.)

Mrs. Taylor, a forty-eight-year-old, attractive, ex-nightclub society singer, was the daughter of Charles Fletcher, one of the town's leading merchants and one of the Four Hundred of Preston. Her husband, a successful criminal lawyer, was a self-made man who had come from the wrong side of the tracks. Mrs. Taylor's warmth and her yen for the romantic were in contrast to her husband, who obviously felt uncomfortable socially and seemed at home only when fighting for his clients. The Taylors had been married for 20 years and had two fine sons — John, nineteen, a premedical student and Charles, fourteen, a high-school student — but their marriage had been a series of fights, with Mr. Taylor occasionally even beating his wife.

Mrs. Taylor had a long medical history and an infinite number of complaints. She had had several D and C's, gastrointestinal x-rays, biliary drainages, and the like. During her frequent visits to the doctor, she spent the greater part of her time complaining about her husband's brutalities and continually talked of divorcing him. Apparently, the Taylors devoted a considerable part of their lives to doing things which infuriated each other.

Finally, Mrs. Taylor left her husband but, when she saw Joe two weeks later, she again had a long list of complaints. She wept through the entire interview and the negative examination. Then she blurted out to Joe that since leaving her husband she had felt "like a flat beer" and had decided to go back to him. Evidently, the Taylors couldn't live with or without each other.

Myron and Mrs. Taylor are people who, of their own volition, pursue a hectic way of life. They want to have their cake and eat it too, that is, they want to live in turmoil but without the distress it necessarily entails. It is impossible to eradicate their symptoms if they continue to live in such a manner. The physician can only point out that peace and serenity are incompatible with their method of existing, and medicine cannot give them peace of mind.

16. DEPRESSION

D R. EVANS felt the futility of his efforts every time he saw Mrs. Arbogast. He had x-rayed her thoroughly, given her belladonna, charcoal, bile salts, and methyl cellulose but her gas, bloating, and constipation persisted. She was getting more tired all the time, could just about drag herself around, and could not sleep without a sedative.

The surgeon was extremely concerned about Mrs. Grace. Before he had performed a mastectomy on her she was a handsome woman, well groomed, socially adept. Now, six weeks after operation, she was not eating, was losing weight, stayed in bed all day, and did not want to leave the hospital. She looked haggard, drawn, and unkempt. She complained of a lot of pain and demanded increasing amounts of narcotics. Her nurse suggested hypodermic injections of sterile water. The surgeon went over her thoroughly and x-rayed her chest again, but could find no evidence of metastases. He told her that the operation was a success, that he had got "it" all out and so on. Parenteral vitamins, high-dosage Vitamin B-12, and a bitter-tasting tonic were likewise of no avail.

Both of these patients were depressed. Mrs. Grace was behaving as if she really had metastatic cancer. When she was allowed and encouraged to talk, she revealed her fears of cancer and her conviction that she was going to die of it. She cried as she talked and this helped her feel better. The fears and fantasies she revealed were answered specifically and effectively. She worried, too, about her appearance and her husband's future feelings toward her. Her appearance was easily improved with a prosthesis. Her husband was told about her scar and her sensitivity; was advised neither to deny the change nor to act shocked about it. Instead the operation and its cosmetic consequences were something to discuss and accept together. After a few sessions, during which Mrs. Grace did most of the talking, she improved quickly — and so did her surgeon.

Mrs. Arbogast was likewise depressed, but her management was different. Joe could have made the diagnosis sooner had he paid more attention to the feelings the patient was engendering in him than to her many complaints. Joe was a good and effective physician and his feelings of therapeutic futility really came from Mrs. Arbogast and her melancholy feelings of worthlessness and hopelessness. When Joe recognized the depression, he learned that Mrs. Arbogast had had two similar episodes in the past ten years with spontaneous recovery each time. He discussed this with the patient and her husband and asked her frankly about the possibility of suicide. She said that although she often thought of it she could be trusted not to carry it out. Joe suggested that no more studies be done. Instead he would support her through this difficult period. Within three months her depression lifted and her symptoms disappeared.

These are but two examples of patients suffering depression. It is a common mood disorder and appears in many guises — often it is manifested in bodily symptoms, especially gastrointestinal ones, insomnia, and fatigue, particularly in the morning. Spontaneous crying and dreams of dead relatives are also common. These findings help substantiate the diagnosis of depression that the physician gets by *feeling* that his patient is "down in the dumps."

It is not intended to discuss in detail this disorder with its broad spectrum of symptoms and its wide variation in severity. However, it is worth emphasizing that:

1. Depression is more common than realized and accounts for many symptoms, particularly those often labeled incorrectly as due to hypometabolism or secondary anemia.

2. Many patients with chronic disease have an accompanying depression that contributes significantly to their disability.

3. If the physician will "up his antenna," he can often sense the patient's depression and use it to guide him in a diagnosis.

Introduction to Chapters 17–21

Dean Brotherston of Edinburgh has expressed fluently the proposition that current medical-school graduates are not shocked or overwhelmed by syphilis and incurable cancer but are often upset about social and emotional disorders. They can tolerate incurable biological illness but are frustrated by incurable social and emotional ills.

These chapters are intended to convey an attitude of tolerance and understanding for those patients who are a diagnostic or therapeutic puzzle, who deny their illness, whose families obstruct medical care, and to illustrate some ways of dealing more effectively with these problems. People are entitled to and will always continue to choose their own way of life. The physician who urges them to choose more wisely should not feel a personal affront if he is ignored, nor should he be angry and reject these people.

17. WISHING WON'T
MAKE IT SO

THE FOLLOWING QUESTION was asked on one of Joe Evans' senior year medical-school examinations:

A sixty-year-old, anxious widow is brought to your office by her married daughter, who informs you that her mother has a lump in her breast, but won't do anything about it. She has been to another doctor who has urged an operation, but she has refused. Her daughter says that her mother has never been one to go to bed when ill.

Outline your handling of this patient.

(Perhaps the reader would be interested in composing his own answer before reading further.)

95

Some of Joe's classmates answered this question in the following manner. After examining the patient they would tell her that she needed hospitalization for tests. They would explain that at first only a small, biopsy *incision* would be made. She would be given adequate *anesthesia* and not suffer *pain*. They would say that the outlook in these lesions caught early, is good. They would explain that not all breast lumps are *cancer* (the italicized words are frightening ones). Other students became angry at this patient. They said that if the measures just mentioned failed, they would tell the patient the cold facts and threaten her with death from spreading cancer if she did nothing about it. One or two were more interested in self-preservation than in patient preservation, and said they would have her sign a release if she refused surgery.

The students who answered as just outlined were in error. They were too active in their management of the patient. They explained, they talked, they exhorted, they entreated, they cajoled, they argued, they threatened. They did not try to understand.

The students who received good grades on this exam realized the importance of understanding that the patient had been fearful all her life. Now, threatened with cancer and a disfiguring operation, she is so frightened that she cannot face the situation. She must deny reality because it is too fearful.

They would encourage her to talk about her fears, to tell of her previous medical experiences, with her husband, parents, and self. They would like to learn from her what she thinks and feels about her future course, her hospitalization. What reasons does she give for not following the doctor's advice? Why does she refuse hospitalization? When her fears and motivations are exposed, there is a good chance that she, herself, will see how fragile they are. The physician, moreover, will have a more precise knowledge of the specific areas for which she needs explanation and reassurance.

This approach has the greatest chance of success in this admittedly difficult situation. It is one of understanding and kindness. It allows the patient to be active, to explain, to talk, probably even to cry.

The physician, meanwhile, has largely limited his part of the conversation to a few questions, why, what, and how does the patient think and feel. The blunderbuss technique, with threats of a dire outcome, is the last resort. If used early, it can so terrify the patient that she may not be able to cooperate. If used at all, it is best saved until last.

In contrast to this situation, the ability to deny

frightening reality can be very much of a blessing in patients with an incurable malignant growth.

A sixty-three-year-old widow had inoperable carcinoma of the head of the pancreas with hepatic metastases. Dr. Evans was called to her home because she was having pain. She was gaunt and wasted, with a large protruding abdomen filled with liver, metastases, and ascites. Surprisingly, she smiled, welcomed Joe warmly, and declared that her operation (an exploratory laparotomy) had helped her greatly. The thing that was bothering her was a hemorrhoid. True, she did have a subacutely thrombosed hemorrhoid which Joe treated vigorously. Obviously, she could not possibly face up to her general condition and needed to displace her concern onto the hemorrhoid. Joe encouraged and supported this displacement.

Most patients with incurable malignant growths use this mechanism of denial. Joe found that even physicians with obvious cancer will talk of infections, vascular disorders and so on, and never mention the word *cancer* or ask about it.

The denial of reality, however, can constitute a real threat to existence. This is especially true of patients with myocardial infarctions who are made so anxious by the disease and by being made to rest in bed, that they find all sorts of excuses to leave the hospital and refuse to restrict their activities. Likewise, some patients with tuberculosis or diabetes find their disease difficult to face and become uncooperative. This attitude sometimes makes the physician so angry that he will threaten the patients with dire results, which may increase their anxiety and result in less — rather than more — cooperation. The approach outlined for the patient with the breast tumor is advocated for patients of this type.

18. THE FAMILY

THE PATIENT'S MIDDLE-AGED HUSBAND made a fine first impression, well groomed, intelligent, and obviously successful. He had remained devotedly with his wife for many trying years, for ever since their marriage she had been sick. When she was physically able she frequented bars and had once been considered a barbiturate addict. She had been taken to many doctors for her alcoholism and drug addiction but none had been of any help. Once she had been admitted to one of the mental hospitals, but her husband signed her out against medical advice, saying "I could not stand to see her in chains." He provided her with a fine home, good clothes, and when she became "nervous" and upset he would dole out a few ounces of whiskey for her. At present she is cachectic, weighing less than 80 pounds, is unable to eat, and has a cirrhotic liver. Her medical condition is precarious.

Eighteen-year-old John Phillips was brought by his parents to Dr. MacDonough for an evaluation of his "epilepsy." They related that he had suffered a grand mal seizure at the age of ten, and since then has had several "seizures," described as staring into space for a few minutes. They had consulted numerous specialists, some of whom urged that John be taken off Dilantin, but his mother refused. She was positive that her boy had epilepsy and needed the medicine, even though the doctors were not. She insisted that he forego swimming, climbing trees, and such for fear of what might happen if he had a seizure. Further investigation revealed that for the past two years he had been failing in school, getting into fights, and had recently beaten up his sister. Studies were negative except for the electroencephalogram which revealed a borderline tracing.

These two patients had serious problems that could not be handled until their families were dealt with first. The husband of the alcoholic was literally killing her with kindness. It was he who negated any positive action that was taken for his wife — he could not stand having her in a mental hospital, could not deprive her of alcohol when she was upset, and so on. Unless he looked at the situation more realistically his wife could die of her alcoholism. His actions may have appeared generous and kindly, but he had to be made to see what his indulgence was doing before she could be given real help.

The case of John also demonstrates a well-meaning but malignant attitude on the part of a family—especially the mother. From his studies, Dr. MacDonough did not believe that the boy had epilepsy, although whether a true grand mal attack occurred at the age of ten can never be absolutely determined. The attack, however, is not the question of the moment. The significant fact is that his mother *insisted* that the boy be treated for epilepsy and blamed all of his aberrant behavior on the fact that he was sick — he had epilepsy. Actually, the boy's major problem was not epilepsy but behavior. The real disease lay in his mother's thinking, her insistence on labeling the boy sick, epileptic, different, all of which has impaired his social growth and maturity. Little can be hoped for him until his mother sees what she is doing.

Some years ago Dr. Evans promised himself that he would advise all parents of retarded children to have them institutionalized. He arrived at this conclusion on having gone to a get-together at the home of a colleague who had three children — a teen-age daughter, a mongoloid child of ten, and a bright young boy of six. The entire family revolved around the defective child — the daughter could not invite her friends to her home because of his antics, the family could not go out because of his unpredictable behavior, and there was little time or energy left for the six-year-old. Joe was appalled by the conditions; four people constantly on edge because of one unfortunate, defective child. His colleague had been advised to have the child placed in a home but had refused, saying he could not and would not.

More recently Joe met a charming matron in her late fifties, the mother of a teen-aged boy with cerebral palsy, who was also mentally defective. The woman had married early and had already raised her family when this last child was born. Despite the seeming hopelessness of his severe handicaps, she spent painstaking hours teaching and caring for the boy. She said that she did not know what she would do with herself if it were not for this child. Such devoted care forced Joe to revise his first rash statement and to realize that, in some diseases, the family is more important than the diagnosis.

19. HUMPTY DUMPTY

*All the King's horses and all the
King's men couldn't put Humpty Dumpty
together again.*

RUTH HIGBY'S FAVORITE EXPRESSION was "Everything happens to me and Dick Tracy." Her younger sister, who was prettier than she, had married well, whereas all that Ruth could catch was a quiet and unprepossessing fellow who worked in a greenhouse. Her brother was highly successful in business and gave his wife everything she desired, but never did anything, according to Ruth, "for his own flesh and blood." One cold day in February, Ruth fell on an icy sidewalk. X-rays of her back were negative but she continued to complain of low-back pain for more than a year. She was studied thoroughly on two occasions by orthopedists, neurosurgeons, gynecologists, and internists without any positive findings. She was not helped by a Camp corset, bedboards, postural correction, exercises, or muscle relaxants.

Joe Evans learned that patients such as Ruth are not uncommon. They usually wander from doctor to doctor, from clinic to clinic, looking for the magical cure, and often wind up in the hands of quacks or charlatans. Their life has been a series of disappointments; has never come up to their expectations. They dream in vain of the better life, are sometimes motion picture or television devotees, gaining a little vicarious happiness from the rags-to-riches stories. When sick or injured, their unhappiness and their hopes become focused on their illness, which becomes the *raison d'être* for their troubles. Doctors and their medicines become their great hope for salvation.

Dr. Evans explained to Ruth the unreality of her ways, pointing out that perhaps she could achieve more of the happiness and even healthiness she desired if she would spend her time, energy, and money striving for some of the ends she wished for, instead of concentrating all of her energies and resources on her illness. Contrary to what Tin Pan Alley says, wishing won't make it so.

Henry Moroni had been falling asleep at odd and embarrassing moments for the past two years. He had seen and been treated without benefit by a number of excellent physicians. Finally, on the recommendation of a friend, he consulted Dr. Chernas, told him of his complaints, and the fact that no one had been able to help him. Chernas said that he wasn't surprised, that psychiatrists didn't help anybody anyhow — they only make people poor. If he was "nuts," he might as well commit himself to the state asylum and save himself a lot of time and money. The patient was indignant. Of course he wasn't crazy and certainly he didn't need an insane asylum — but what could he do? "Stop falling asleep," Chernas answered. "What are you, a child that needs a nap every day?" The patient was taken aback. "You mean," he stammered, "it's up to me?" "Sure," said Chernas, "it's up to you." The patient has slept only at night ever since.

One of Joe Evans' most frustrating patients was Sammy Fox, a boy of ten. The child, who had come along seven years after his next older sibling and was the baby of the family, had a history of a sore throat followed by pain in the right wrist. The initial diagnosis of rheumatic fever was disproved after three weeks of thorough study in a children's hospital. The boy, however, continued to complain, especially of pain in the wrist and knee. He could not write because of pain in the wrist and could not walk because of pain and weakness in the knee. He was recommended to a large number of expert physicians and

was studied extensively in a university hospital. He
and his mother were told that he did or did not
have rheumatic fever, Still's disease, or lupus
erythematosus. His studies included innumerable
blood counts and urinalyses, several electrocardiograms, x-rays of every organ available to this instru-
ment, plasma electrophoresis, several histological
tests for lupus erythematosus, an electroencephalogram, and a BMR. He had been treated with several
of the latest steroids, salicylates in high dosage,
p-aminobenzoic acid, and so on, to no avail. After
three years of such studies the family had exhausted
most of its funds and their son had not been out of
the house, except to visit physicians and hospitals. His
schooling had to be carried on by a private teacher,
he had no social life, and, at thirteen years of age,
was a shut-in with no objective physical findings. It
was at this point that his mother brought Sammy to
Joe Evans.

After a review of the patient's extensive records,
Joe asked the boy's mother what she wanted. "I want,"
she said, "a definite diagnosis, an end to the confusion.
I want to know why the doctors can't agree as to just
what disease my boy has. I want somebody to get my
son better." The mother was disconcerted when Joe
told her that he didn't know what the diagnosis was,
that he wasn't going to do any more tests to find out,

that the precise diagnosis was not his primary concern. She was wasting time and money looking further
for "the" diagnosis. She had been doing this for years
and where did it get her? She had seen the best
physicians and they weren't sure; certainly, Joe had
no more talent, no more diagnostic magic than they.
She had been pursuing the pot of gold at the end
of the rainbow, and it just wasn't there. All the
diagnostic studies and all the medicines had not
made her son better. To keep going this way meant
hopeless invalidism for her son. Joe Evans held out,
instead, a hopeful future. He was concerned with
Sammy's disability. Was he to live, to grow up, to go
to school, to marry? If so, the only course left was
for him to begin to live despite the lack of a diagnosis.

At this point, Sammy became furious. He screamed
at Dr. Evans, swore that his was real pain and that he
was really sick (Joe had never said otherwise). He
cursed all doctors, and Joe agreed that he had cause
to be angry with them. Joe pointed out that he was
sure that Sammy did not want to be an invalid all
his life, to be always a second-rate citizen. The boy
replied by demanding with screams and sobs that
Joe get rid of his pain. Joe said he would do his best
to help him, see that he did not "get hurt," that he
was in no danger, and that he must be a very
frightened boy. When Sammy calmed down, Joe

asked him about school work. The boy said he
couldn't write because of the pain in his right wrist.
Joe asked why he didn't try to write left-handed? He
had tried, he replied, but his left hand got too tired!
That was important information. It confirmed Joe's
impression that this boy's disability was not due to
his pains or to his "disease"; instead, it indicated that
the child was afraid of school, of the world, of
growing up.

Again the boy's mother insisted on a "real"
diagnosis. (So did the hospital staff later on when the
case was presented to them.) Joe reiterated that his
chief concern was with the child's disability. He
offered hope that the boy could grow and develop,
that time need not stand still until a precise diagnosis
was established. Then the mother asked if her son
should see a psychiatrist. Joe said that this again
was pursuing the magic cure — another doctor, another diagnosis. He felt that administering psychotherapy at this time would not be basically different
from administering prednisone. No one had made
the boy better. It was up to Sammy himself to begin
to reduce his own disability. Of course, Joe knew
that a great deal of work for him remained to be
done with this patient and his mother, but a way
out of an insoluble diagnostic quandary had been
opened. When the boy began to reduce his own disa-

bility, when he would talk about himself, his fears, and anger, would be time enough for him to work *with* a psychiatrist on his problem. Moreover the rapport gained from improvement would facilitate a psychiatric referral. Presently any implication that the problem was emotional would likely force the family to strengthen their defenses against the real nature of the problem.

Privately Joe warned the mother that her boy might have an exacerbation of his symptoms in the coming week, that he might feel a need to demonstrate his sickness and helplessness. The symptoms did recur but the mother was prepared for them and did not become alarmed. On the next visit, Sammy was sullen but admitted he had gone out of the house and had walked two blocks. Joe was profuse in his praise of this accomplishment. The following week, Sammy and his mother went shopping downtown and bought clothing. Joe was exultant and let the boy know how proud he was of him. But disappointment followed; Sammy did not come for his next visit. On calling the boy's home, Joe learned that the boy had been sent to another hospital for further study.

Joe often thought about this case and wondered if he could not have done better. Should he have pursued further diagnostic studies? No, he decided, he had been right to emphasize the disability aspects and minimize the disease. It still seemed the only way out of a bad situation.

Disease and disability are not the same. The physician's eye must be on the sparrow as well as on the injured wing.

20. YOU ARE NOT SICK

ONE DAY Joe Evans was asked for advice by Jane Brown, his next-door neighbor. Mrs. Brown, whom the Evanses had known for several years, was always well thought of in the community. She was the mother of four children, the youngest six months old. Her husband was a lawyer who had had considerable difficulty with alcoholism during the past two years, with periods when he had been unable to work and episodes of abusiveness to his wife. Despite these difficulties, Mrs. Brown quietly kept the family going and things did seem a little improved lately.

Mrs. Brown told Joe that during her last pregnancy, she had had some abdominal distress which she had tried to ignore, believing it to be part of the discomfort of pregnancy. When the pain persisted after delivery, she reported it to her physician. X-rays disclosed suggestive evidence of a peptic ulcer whereupon her physician put her on a bland antacid diet. He scolded her for getting upset and told her that she would have to stop worrying.

Jane Brown was ashamed of her ulcer. She had been a psychology major in college and believed the illness was an indication of personal weakness. Since her physician had advised her not to keep things to herself, she asked Joe if it really would do any good for her to scream at the children? She feared it would only hurt them. What should she do? Was she neurotic? Did he think she needed psychiatric treatment?

This was the first time Joe had ever seen Mrs. Brown so upset and anxious. After a bit of rapid thinking, he pointed out that with all that she had been through she had handled herself extremely well and had been very stable. Was all the concern she was now manifesting about the alleged ulcer really a reaction to all the trouble she had borne? How about her feelings of anxiety and concern over her husband? Were they pathological — is that what she learned in her psychology courses? It seemed clear to him that it would be pathological if she didn't feel anxious. He also differed with the physician who told her "not to worry." In Joe's mind that only added one more worry to the long list she already had.

He concluded the conversation with some ideas he had on the causes of peptic ulcers. To the best of his knowledge, he said, it had never been absolutely proved that emotions cause ulcers. The role of emotions was still hypothetical and the majority of ulcers could be managed quite well on a medical regimen.

Jane Brown thanked Joe and said she felt relieved. She would do her best to handle whatever came her way — it was foolish to be so upset over an ulcer which she might have — she had enough real problems to keep her hands full.

21. THE PROBLEM
OF MEDICAL DISABILITY

IT HAS BEEN ESTIMATED that one person in six is medically disabled and the amount of time, money, and energy spent in trying to remedy this situation by medical means is staggering. The real cause of much so-called "medical" disability is to be found in our highly developed technological society, where the demand for the unskilled worker is low and automation is making obsolete many skills of the recent past. Unless these displaced workers can learn new trades, they are without jobs and income. Industry, labor, and even the worker himself sometimes find "medical" disability the undisputed way out of this dilemma. "Medical" disability can and often does constitute a medical solution for a social problem.

Mary Yancey was one of Dr. Chernas' favorite

people. She had been his valued and dependable housekeeper for ten years, as well as his patient. Since the birth of her last child, he had treated her intermittently for high blood pressure which ranged from 164/100 to 180/120. Despite his frequent admonishments to stop working so hard — she even used to cut the lawn — Mary always declared that work was good for a body and kept working. She had a difficult home situation which Dr. Chernas helped with as best he could — her husband was a loafer who drank a lot and never held a steady job. Mary had been practically the sole support of her five children. Knowing how industrious she had always been, Dr. Chernas was astonished when she told him that she had been unable to work and had been on public assistance for the past year. She asked him to sign her yearly slip certifying her to be medically disabled from high blood pressure. Dr. Chernas asked what had happened. Mary confided that four of the children had grown up, married, and left home. Her youngest, now eighteen, had turned out to be a bad boy who periodically got into trouble with the police and was forever demanding money from her. He was just like her husband, who was still taking whatever money he could find for liquor. At this point Mary broke down and cried — she just couldn't work any longer, she had headaches, felt dizzy, was just too sick.

This case illustrates some of the many facets of the problem of medical disability. In such situations it is the patient who states that he is disabled and unable to work. The physician then must state why (hypertension). Mary had had hypertension for years and actually worked beyond medical recommendations. Yet, after most of her family had grown, the futility of slaving for a shiftless husband and a no-good son made it impossible for her to continue. She then collapsed with a multitude of complaints.

Frequently the actual physical condition of the person has little or nothing to do with the disability itself. Because Dr. Chernas had known Mary, he understood the real problem and the source of her disability. He appreciated the futility of trying to get her off the welfare roles by curing her hypertension or removing her symptoms by direct treatment. Another physician, unaware of the whole situation, may have accepted the hypertension as the "real" cause of her disability and given her medical sanction to be unemployed until cured of her disease. This iatrogenic factor is common in chronic disability.

Greg Bascombe had always been fleshy and still was. The only boy of five children, he had always been pampered by his mother and sisters. After barely graduating from high school, Greg got a job as a clerk and worked at it uninspiredly for five years. One day, when he was in the company shop, a workman dropped a heavy forging on Greg's foot and fractured it. Two years later, Greg was still on crutches. X-rays and examination of the foot were negative, but Greg said that it was painful to walk on and that it would not bear his weight. He was advised to lose weight but how could he when he could not get around and be active because of his foot? Two of Greg's sisters called the doctor on several occasions, demanding to know exactly what was wrong with his foot and insisting that the doctor do something. They offered to pay the expenses of sending him to some other specialist. A lawyer heard of Greg and persuaded him to sue the company on a contingency basis for $20,000. He claimed that damages were due Greg for the fracture, the hospital and doctors' bills, the loss of income, the pain and sufferings, and the fact that Greg had to postpone his proposed wedding indefinitely because he was unable to support a wife.

Our system of compensation pays people who are disabled and nonproductive, the amount of payment varying directly with the degree of disability. Some people can spend years, just as Greg has, feeling that they have been wronged by fate and deserve to collect disability payments. They devote their time to proving how disabled they are instead of concentrating their efforts on becoming able again. Of course, as long as people receive gain from what they cannot do, this situation will be present.

The eventual outcome of cases like Greg's, unfortunately, is that physicians become angry at the patients and decide that their problem is "all in the head." At this rather late stage they are "rejected to" a psychiatrist in the hope that he will be able to push the right button and set them to working again. The psychiatrist, on the other hand, is faced with a patient who has come in against his will, who asserts adamantly that his trouble is physical and not imaginary, and who wouldn't undergo treatment if Sigmund Freud himself offered it free of charge. In this spot, the psychiatrist may find that all he can do is apply a diagnostic label, such as "passive dependent personality." This evaluation does not relieve the situation for two reasons. The first is that this is the same thing that occurred with Mary Yancey. The patient states that he cannot work, and the physician applies some diagnostic label, this time a psychiatric one. The second reason is that everyone has a personality pattern of some kind, and for every passive dependent person who is not working there are hundreds who are working. The psychiatrist usually finds himself as therapeutically impotent in this situation as is everyone else.

One possible way of approaching a problem such as Greg's is:

DOCTOR: The examination of your foot is negative. I wonder why you don't go back to work?

GREG: But it still hurts to walk on and it's weak
and it swells up, and . . .

DOCTOR: Greg, I believe that actions speak louder
than words and, if this is so, one might question
if you really are interested in returning to work.

GREG: Of course, I really am, but my foot . . .

DOCTOR: I keep telling you that you're okay and
you keep arguing that you are not. It seems as
if you are spending all your time proving you are
sick, instead of following my advice and going
back to work — even in spite of your foot.

GREG: But I have tried to walk on it and it hurts.

DOCTOR: So?

GREG: The pain . . .

DOCTOR: You know, Greg, whether you work or
you don't is up to you. I have recommended repeatedly that you *try* but you haven't — so that
neither of us knows for sure if you can. I do know
that the chances of your returning to work are nil
unless you do try. I have seen many patients who
have been unsure of themselves about improving
— whose entire life becomes centered around a

symptom. They say that if only they didn't have this symptom all would be well — but they *do* have it. The price of *not* trying is very high — it is almost as if one has to dedicate his life to proving to himself and others that he can't work.

We have done all that can be done about the pain — perhaps you can learn to live with it.

When it seems to the patient that continued disability is to his advantage, it is probable that no technique will alter the situation, but the facts should be stated honestly. Moreover, in our opinion, the diagnostic label has little to do with the disability; there are cardiacs who work, passive-dependents who work, psychotics who work, and paraplegics who work, despite their diagnosis. This realization seems highly significant when one considers the constant increases in social security and veterans' benefits, workmen's compensation, and other disability payments.

Introduction to Chapters 22–24

The two questions most frequently asked by patients and their families are: (1) what is it? and (2) how long will it last? Medical education must necessarily be aimed at answering the first question, that is, at making the diagnosis and understanding the disease. The second question is often more difficult to answer and even if answered must be less precise. Technical phrases such as "the prognosis is guarded" or "it is a disease of remissions and exacerbations" have little meaning to the layman. Knowing the natural history of a disease is basic to medical understanding, yet interindividual variations often make accurate prediction impossible. Even if prognosticating could be more precise the sensitive physician must be concerned with the impact of the "facts" about a disorder on the feelings of the patient and his family. Art and feeling must accompany science.

22. THE CRYSTAL BALL

THE PROFESSOR OF CARDIOLOGY, a wise and gentle man, had advised Joe and his classmates in medical school never to venture a prognosis to the patient or to his family. At the time this suggestion did not impress Joe particularly. He had the assurance of the inexperienced, and almost every other lecturer ended his exposition of a disorder with "prognosis." With the hindsight of a few years in practice, however, Joe formulated his own rules: (1) a pessimistic prognosis, even if correct, can cause a great deal of unnecessary anguish and (2) an optimistic prognosis, even if eventually incorrect, can bring considerable relief to a harrassed patient and his family. He decided that the scientific accuracy of a prediction, although important, is not the single determinant but the therapeutic effect is a

most significant value. Joe agreed with his old professor that no prognosis at all was often better than
a gloomy one. He could not agree, however, that all
prognoses should be avoided, for a favorable prognosis, even though eventually wrong, could often
serve a humane and therapeutic purpose.

During his first year in practice, Joe had a young
couple who brought their infant son and only child
for routine pediatric care. The boy seemed to thrive,
but Joe noted and the parents remarked upon his
unusually large head. When his fontanelles did not
close at the proper time, Joe had skull x-rays taken.
The radiologist agreed with the possibility of early
hydrocephalus but could not be sure. Joe felt impelled to tell the baby's parents of his diagnosis and
to warn them of the possible future difficulties they
faced. They were shocked and disbelieving. He next
saw the family a year later when they met accidentally.
The parents showed the boy defiantly, told Joe how
well he was doing, and said that they had taken him
to a pediatrician who denied that he had "water on
the brain." Joe noticed that, although the boy looked
well, he still had a large head, and he wondered if the
child would have future cerebral difficulties.

In retrospect, however, Joe realized that the accuracy or inaccuracy of his diagnosis was not the
important issue. He had caused these parents a great

deal of concern at a time when no one could have done anything about the possible disorder. It would have been much better to keep his concerns to himself, to watch the child carefully, and to wait. He knew that the pediatrician, too, must have had some private doubts and consequently admired the latter's optimism all the more.

When Morris Levin was sixty-four he complained to Joe of a substernal pain on exertion, typical of angina pectoris. His electrocardiogram was grossly abnormal. Joe thought the outlook was poor and confided this to the patient's wife. "About 20 percent of such patients die suddenly," he warned. The patient, now seventy-four years of age, was still coming to see Joe regularly with occasional pain. Joe realized that his prophecies of doom had been of no help either to the patient or to his wife and that she had been living in dread for ten years. He knew, too, that his pessimistic prognosis had been motivated in part by his own fear of being criticized if his patient did not do well. Self-concern, rather than patient-concern, had induced him to voice his dismal, albeit statistically accurate, prediction. A doctor of medicine ought to be big enough to take such risks, he decided.

Joe discussed these ideas with Dr. MacDonough, who expressed his own concern that physicians would be criticized for not telling the truth about a patient's future. As they considered the problem, however, it became clear that the truth was often uncertain and unknown, especially in the area of prognosis. It was true enough to state that Morris Levin had coronary artery disease, but the prediction of imminent death was inaccurate in his particular case. MacDonough recalled a number of patients who did much better than statistical probabilities had suggested, one of whom was a young man with Hodgkins disease, who, treated several times with x-ray irradiation, was now, 15 years later, apparently cured. He told of how he had worried when this young man's wife continued to have babies every year because as a doctor, he believed the patient would not live long.

Dr. Evans and Dr. MacDonough concluded that their ability to predict the course of a disease was limited and that, for the individual patient, mortality statistics were of little use. "Truth" was an area of wide latitude and, in prognosticating, one must make his own base from which to decide what to say and how to say it.

Joe often thought to himself that people's future behavior was actually more predictable than the course of their disease.

23. THE PLACE
FOR PESSIMISM

S HORTLY AFTER THESE CONVERSATIONS Joe and
Sally Evans received an invitation to the
MacDonough's. The two men withdrew to the
study, where Mac offered Joe some bourbon and then
began to talk on his favorite topic — medicine. It was
obvious that he enjoyed talking with Joe and felt
some paternal interest in moderating Joe's youthful
enthusiasm. He said that although he agreed with
Joe's ideas on optimism in diagnosis and prognosis
he did think that there was also a place for pessimism.

Mac recalled a family whose seventy-year-old bedridden mother was a cantankerous, irascible creature
who irritated everyone. Numerous physicians had
been called in and then discharged when they were

not able to improve the old lady's condition and behavior significantly. Dr. MacDonough said that after
he was called into the case he was plagued by phone
calls from every member of the family, asking him
what he thought, suggesting what he should do, and
recommending consultations with various specialists.
Actually, he said, everything that could be done was
already being done — there was simply nothing more
that medicine had to offer. Dr. MacDonough decided
to call a meeting of the entire family. He told them
that he understood their anxiety and admired their
concern for their mother but explained that she was
not going to change for the better, no matter what
was done. If for no other reason than for their own
peace and happiness, the time had come to put their
mother in a nursing home. It was time to face it —
stop searching for miracles, abandon the hysteria,
and act like mature people.

"Optimism, Joe, would certainly have been out of
place in this situation — pessimism, or perhaps the
better word is realism, was appropriate."

Joe then told of one of his cases which confirmed
Mac's ideas. A twelve-year-old boy, thought by his
mother to have epilepsy, was constantly moving about,
blinking his eyes, contorting his face, posturing his
limbs. Joe was unable to find any definite neuro-
logical findings. An electroencephalogram was at-

tempted but was unsuccessful because the boy could not sit still. The picture did not fit either Sydenham's or Huntington's chorea but the boy was obviously a "nervous wreck." He was the youngest of four siblings, the others all normal. Early in his schooling he was found to be mentally retarded and was placed in special classes. His mother then devoted herself to teaching him and spent many hours a day going over his lessons, drilling him in spelling, and so on. Twice a week special tutors came to the house, even during summer vacations in a constant effort to improve the boy's mind.

It was not easy, but Joe had to tell the mother that her well-intended efforts were futile. Her boy simply did not have the mentality to overcome his handicap and be like normal children. It was unfortunate but true. Could she love him for what he was — protect him, support him, but give up her efforts to improve him? The boy could not cope with all that was being asked of him and it was these demands that were causing his great "nervousness" and peculiar behavior. This situation, too, called for pessimism in prognosis.

24. NEVER UNDERESTIMATE
THE POWER OF ...

ONE DAY, while walking down the street, Joe bumped into Mrs. Peggy Bigelow. He failed to recognize her at first because she was now a charming, vibrant matron of forty-five obviously in the flower of health. When he was able to collect his wits, Joe asked her to what she attributed this miracle. She smiled pleasantly, answered "good living," and continued on her way.

Joe remembered Mrs. Bigelow only too well. She had what was probably the largest medical chart in the county. She had been the bane of many physicians — one of those patients with everything in the books, including the complications. She had seen several psychiatrists and had had numerous psychiatric hospitalizations — Joe knew of two for alcoholism and one for attempted suicide. She had been disgruntled and petulant with little regard for the medical profession or anyone else. Her long-suffering husband, almost twenty years her senior, looked after her as if she were a wayward child. They themselves were childless, so that he seemed to dedicate much of his time to helping her, always careful not to concern her with problems or worries. Her reaction to his solicitude was continual complaining and grumbling. Her behavior when drinking was so unpredictable and unpleasant that they lost all their friends. Joe knew her as irritable, spoiled, and thoroughly miserable; he could not believe the change.

Later he learned the explanation for the miracle. Her husband was found to have severe diabetes and for the first time in her married life she had a responsibility. She prepared his meals, checked the correctness of his diet, supervised his medication, drove him to work, and was even able to help him in his small business. One afternoon on his way home from work her husband went into shock from an insulin reaction and was taken to the hospital. Not knowing where he was until that evening, she had become frantic with worry. The next day she became psychotic — hallucinating, rambling, out of contact — and had to be hospitalized. In just five days, however, she recovered and demanded to be discharged because she had to take care of her husband. On past occasions, she would have been a patient for a month or longer. She still could not stand much stress, but with a purpose in life her recuperative power was amazing.

Joe learned that unforseen events can produce unpredictable changes for better or for worse in a patient. His respect heightened for the cardiology professor who had counseled care in making prognoses.

25. THE UNCERTAIN DIAGNOSIS

JOE MET DR. MAC DONOUGH a short time later in the Staff Room at Memorial Hospital. Mac said that he had been thinking of Joe's rules of prognosis and felt that they might apply also to diagnosis in some instances. For example, a jittery, chain-smoking, young laborer with a wife and three small children was sent to him complaining of chest pain. A fellow-worker had died on the job and was known to have had a bad heart and the patient was afraid he would suffer a similar fate. After a careful history, Mac could not be sure whether angina was truly present. The physical examination was normal except for generalized hyperactive reflexes; the electrocardiograms were borderline.

135

Noting the kind of nervous person he was, Mac told the patient that he did not have heart disease. He said that there was nothing wrong with his heart by any of the tests. He did not qualify his statements in any way, as, for example, by saying "Let me check you again in six months." He took this position, aware that he might be wrong and that the patient might conceivably drop dead on the job. He believed, however, that the diagnosis was uncertain and that there was no reasonable way in which to make it definitive. But to tell the patient of his uncertainty or to diagnose his pain as heart disease would be to disable him and pauperize his family. For the good of them all, Mac said, "I stuck my neck out and told him he had no heart disease and no physical limitations."

Joe agreed with Dr. MacDonough's decision but posed two questions. Suppose that the patient had gone to another physician, who told him (1) that he definitely had coronary heart disease and that he needed to come to him once a week for treatment or (2) that he, the physician, did not know whether the patient had such heart disease but thought that the patient must assess the future risks and decide whether to continue to work or give it up.

MacDonough quickly disposed of the second possibility. He said that such a physician was shirking his personal responsibility: "Might as well hand the electrocardiogram to the patient and ask him to read it, as ask him to decide on his own diagnosis and treatment." To the first possibility, Mac grunted, "Would have to be a damned quack to make that diagnosis." When calmer, he decided that it was a risk he would have to run and that fortunately his reputation was good enough to withstand it. For legal reasons, he said he had made good notes in the patient's chart, both about the findings and about the reasons for his management. He still believed that he had made the right decision.

Joe recalled a similar situation in which he had decided to be optimistic about the diagnosis to prevent disabling his patient. She was the fifteen-year-old daughter of two intelligent parents, who had become concerned about their daughter's shyness, her disinclination toward parties (especially boy-girl parties), her complete lack of interest in dating. They wanted her to enjoy the country club, to swim, to play tennis, and to meet the "right boys." She seemed, however, much more interested in books than in boys. They took her to a psychologist for testing and were shaken when he reported "obsessive day-dreaming, latent homosexuality, and schizoid tendencies." After a hush-hush consultation with Joe and inquiries about a good psychoanalyst, they brought in the daughter for Joe to meet.

Joe found that she was a bit heavy and suffering
from mild acne. She was shy and quiet in contrast with
her bright and quick mother. Joe spoke to her about
her reading, found her to be quite intelligent and
rather introspective. He liked her and felt sorry for
her. He knew, too, that to label her schizoid and a
latent homosexual could stigmatize her for life. First
he warned her parents not to say a word of this to
anyone, for no mother in Preston would let her child
associate with a "schiz," much less a homosexual, and
the girl would be more isolated than ever. Then he
stated that he disagreed with the psychological assessment. Everyone daydreamed, he said, especially at
that age. Everyone went through a stage of greater
interest in the same sex than in the opposite sex. He
asked her father if he remembered the days of his
early boyhood when girls were terrible creatures,
especially sisters, and didn't the mother remember
when boys were "snakes and snails and puppy dogs'
tails?"

Joe told them that he did not think their daughter
was sick — certainly not schizophrenic. He wondered
if the parents, in their natural desire to see her do
well, had not set too ambitious standards of their own
for their daughter. Perhaps she had different likes and
dislikes, different ideas. Certainly they did not make
her sick. He suggested that they praise her good

qualities, try to overlook her faults, not push her too hard and, finally, send her away to college. The family, however, still felt strongly that a psychiatric consultation was in order. Joe referred them to the psychiatrist at University whom he had met in the Functional Clinic. The latter reported that the girl was using intellectual defenses against her problems of growing up but that the prognosis was good. He suggested that Dr. Evans follow her periodically to assess future need for psychotherapy. He wondered if a mature social worker was available for counseling.

A few years later the same patient came to Joe's office with her intended husband for a premarital examination. He was tall, thin, wore glasses, and needed a haircut. He was studying for his Ph.D., she said. She apologized for not asking Dr. and Mrs. Evans to their wedding. "Mother wanted a big reception at the club, but I insisted on a small one, just immediate family, you know." Joe knew that his plan of management had worked well, but whether it had or had not, an optimistic diagnosis had been the right thing to offer in this circumstance.

26. DEATH, DYING,
AND DIGNITY

J OE EVANS sat pensively in his office. For a man
who had just saved a life, he did not feel at all
elated; were there times when it was better not
to save a life?

Joe had admitted Mrs. Janet Smith to the hospital
two months previously for a carcinoma of the uterine
fundus with extensive metastases including involvement of the spinal cord. Two weeks after admission
she had tried to take her life by slashing her anesthetic
left leg with a razor. She had cut it to the bone. It
had taken heroic work on the part of almost the entire hospital staff to save her life. Twenty-two pints
of blood and precision teamwork by many physicians
and nurses had accomplished the miracle. Today,

properly repentant, she was being sent to a nursing
home to spend her few remaining bedridden weeks
or months awaiting the final scourge of her relentless
cancer.

Joe was not an advocate of euthanasia. He believed
that a physician must be on the side of life lest he
incur the possibility of a devastating public distrust.
He wondered, though, in the case of a patient like
Janet Smith, if the physician was prolonging life or
prolonging death? He knew of a physician, in charge
of an artificial kidney, who had been pressed into
treating a few patients with terminal glomerulone-
phritis. This man did not believe that he had saved
a life, but that his treatment had caused the patients
to die twice. Inquiring about the moral aspects, Joe
learned that the major religions agreed that a physician was not obligated to use "unusual measures" to
save truly suffering patients with incurable, terminal
diseases. Intravenous fluids were considered "unusual
measures." Joe found this attitude reasonable and
helpful, but nevertheless thought it wise to err on the
side of life.

George Stone consulted Joe because of dissatisfaction with his previous physician. He said he
wanted to see someone whose treatment was more consistent with his own wishes. Joe was shocked by Mr.
Stone's straightforward criticism of his past medical

management and his demand to know Joe's recommendations before engaging him. His first impulse
was to express righteous indignation at the audacity
of a patient challenging the wisdom of his physician's
therapy, but he learned from experience that to act on
first impressions was of little help; he decided to hear
the patient out.

George Stone was one of Preston's leading citizens,
universally respected for his industry, fair play, and
common sense. He was an active participant in many
civic activities as well as President of Stone Industries,
one of the largest companies in the community. Mr.
Stone complained of a "little heart trouble" for the
past two years. The previous summer, while on va-
cation, he had suffered a coronary occlusion and had
spent two months hospitalized in a distant city. He was
on digitalis, occasional injections of a mercurial di-
uretic, and nitroglycerine. His physician had insisted
that he stop working, ordered him to quit his civic
activities, greatly limited his physical activity, put
him on a salt-free, low-fat diet, demanded that he
give up smoking, and asked him to take a two-hour
rest in the afternoon and be in bed by nine in the evening. He could watch television, but not the fights. He
was to avoid all disputes and tensions.

George Stone was frank in speaking of his condition. He realized that his heart was in poor shape but

said he would rather "go with his boots on." He had
been on the suggested regimen for a number of
months but just could not continue, stating causti-
cally, "I don't know whether this will help me live
longer." He assured Joe that all his affairs were in
order and that he wished to continue doing what he
reasonably could as long as he could. He had seen
too many of his friends "killed by retiring."

Although the first physician's recommendations
were in keeping with the patient's objective findings,
it was obvious that his restrictions were more than the
patient could or would bear. The regimen was sci-
entifically correct but not tailored to this particular
person. Joe accepted Mr. Stone as a patient and soon
found that he, too, had joined with the many who admired and respected him.

Jessie Trailor was found semiconscious in her
apartment and was sent to the Emergency Room of
Community Hospital. A widow of seventy-two, she
had lived alone for years on a meager pension. Her
only child, a successful businessman, lived in another
city. Some said it was shameful how he neglected his
mother; others defended him by saying it was the
only thing he could do.

Joe arranged for her admission to a ward where
she could be given the necessary care. The son was

notified and several days later came to see his mother. He went into a rage, demanded a private room and private nurses, wanted to call in his own physician and several specialists. Joe, as calmly as he could, described the situation. The mother was in poor condition, run down, apparently had not been eating well, but everything possible was now being done for her. Joe could not hide his own anger at the son, knowing that the woman would not have been in such a desperate situation if her son had shown any previous interest in her. When Mrs. Trailor died her son threatened to sue Joe for malpractice. Although he never actually did, he wrote to the hospital and the County Medical Society listing his complaints, causing Joe some trouble and embarrassment.

Looking back on it later, Joe realized that he might have handled the situation better. When Mr. Trailor descended on Preston demanding the "most that money could buy" for his mother, Joe should have foreseen possible difficulties. It seemed that Mr. Trailor, feeling guilty for having neglected his mother, suddenly had to make it all up. When Joe intimated that the whole thing might not have happened had he been a more attentive son, Mr. Trailor had no alternative but to blame Joe and thus appease his own conscience. The fact that Joe had seen Mrs. Trailor periodically and administered to her needs for little or no recompense did not entitle him to this attitude toward her son — at least, he should not have voiced it aloud.

It was eleven o'clock on a sweltering summer night when Joe received an emergency call from the family of a patient of Dr. Chernas, a man of seventy who recently had had two myocardial infarctions. The patient's wife, son, and daughter-in-law, disappointed that Dr. Chernas was not available, crowded into the steaming bedroom with Joe where he found the patient *in extremis.* Joe's first impulse was to ask the family to leave but, realizing that the patient was going to die momentarily, he ordered each of the family members to massage an extremity vigorously toward the heart, while he administered a variety of vasopressors and cardiac stimulants. After an appropriate interval, he pronounced the patient dead.

When Dr. Chernas saw Joe the next day, he thanked him for his kindness to the family who said they knew that "everything had been done."

One day Joe was approached by the intern on private medicine who indignantly asked, "Why don't we quit the malarkey about infection and tell Mr. Strauss honestly that he has cancer? He put me on the spot again today, asking if we found anything." Isaac Strauss had been in the hospital for three weeks and studies indicated that his bronchogenic carcinoma was beyond hope. Joe replied by asking the intern if he thought that any intelligent person in the United States who had smoked two to three packs of cigarettes a day for years, had lost thirty pounds, and had a progressive cough and hemoptysis did not *know* he had cancer? The intern answered that yes a person should know, but if he knew, why would he keep asking? Joe could not answer this but pointed out that Mr. Strauss, according to his wife, had put all of his business affairs in order before coming to the hospital. "He knew the diagnosis before we did," Joe remarked. Then he added, "If you really want to cheer him up, go in and play a little gin rummy with him, but watch out that you don't lose your shirt. When he was well he would rather play gin than eat."

27. INSTANT DIAGNOSIS

THE ABILITY to get to the core of the problem does not necessarily depend on voluminous material or lengthy observation. The following cases demonstrate the speed with which one can arrive at the significant aspects of a problem.

1. The young wife of a sailor in the regular Navy is brought to the accident dispensary because she is hysterical. Her husband has just left for extended sea duty.

Has she more to gain by her hysteria than by a cure? Has her husband been returned to shore duty in the past because of her outbursts? If so, little can be done to help her until she accepts the necessity of his sea duty.

2. A policeman is hospitalized for chest pains re-

sulting from an automobile accident while on duty.
Despite four hospitalizations during the past year, no
definite diagnosis has been made and no pathological
process discovered.

Does this case involve litigation? If so, little can be
done until the legal aspect is settled. It might be
pointed out that the patient is spending his time and
energy proving that he is disabled, rather than in re-
habilitating himself.

3. A shabbily clothed mother of eight children complains in the clinic of aches and pains in almost every
system of her body.

Is she on public assistance? If so, she needs to re-
main disabled in order to eat.

4. An attractive young woman complains of frigid-
ity and of dyspareunia so severe she fears it will break
up her marriage.

What is the status of the general marital relationship? When a marriage is failing, dyspareunia is a frequent complaint. It has the advantage of being a
medical problem and, therefore, relieves the patient
from acknowledging an interpersonal problem. Unless
the marital relationship improves, the chances of
curing the dyspareunia are remote.

5. A forty-two-year-old engineer, seeking psychiatric help, is sure that his rheumatoid arthritis is caused by emotional problems. There has been increasingly severe deformity.

Is he, out of desperation, looking for a miraculous cure? Psychiatry may be of help if there are areas of life which the patient is not handling well, but to imply that psychiatric help will cure the arthritis is incorrect. If the arthritis is due, in part, to emotional factors, it conceivably could be helped by improving the patient's general attitude, but such help must be considered a bonus.

6. A sixty-four-year-old childless widow with metastatic carcinoma of the breast has generalized aches and pains, insomnia, and loss of appetite. Although without evidence of further metastatic involvement, she is becoming increasingly more dependent on and demanding of her physician.

Is her problem one of being alone and the fear of dying alone? Is there someone nearby whom she can call? Does she have a telephone by her bedside? The possibility of a nursing home should be considered. Discussion of her fears, provision of a bedside phone, and permission to call whenever necessary may brighten her outlook and diminish her complaints.

7. A middle-aged hypertensive man, usually un-
perturbed about his disorder, insists on being seen
although the office schedule is crowded. He is complaining of a frontal headache and the office nurse
does not think it serious enough to deserve prompt
consideration on a busy day.

As his request is out of character, is something different happening or does he *fear* that something is
happening? Does he fear that the headache is the beginning of a stroke? See him!

8. A traveling salesman calls and wants to be examined the same day. He has a small infected pimple
in the pubic region.

Is he really concerned about having a venereal
disease? A few questions about his recent sexual
activities would indicate whether reassurance or a
serologic test is indicated.

9. An unmarried man complains that he smells
bad and covers his mouth with his hand when talking to you at close range. You smell his breath and it
is not offensive.

Does he feel that people are avoiding him or talking
about his problem behind his back? He shows a symptom characteristic of that of a paranoid schizophrenic.

10. A seventy-three-year-old widow is brought to the office because of preoccupation with a sexual indiscretion in her late teens. She is very distressed.

What is the present-day reality situation that needs attention? Dwelling on some past indiscretion frequently indicates unsolved problems in the present. This particular patient is living with her daughter, son-in-law, and three young children in a small house. She feels unwanted and fears that she is an added burden to her already overworked daughter.

11. A widower, sixty-five years old, married his thirty-five-year-old housekeeper and fathered a child. At the age of seventy he had a stroke which left him with a left hemiplegia. Despite an excellent recovery he complains bitterly of various pains and his inability to function as in the past. He is exceedingly irritable with his wife, who is working part time.

Is this man in need of more physiotherapy, papaverine, anticoagulants, or what? Actually his problem is sexual impotency since the stroke. He fears that his young wife will seek this pleasure elsewhere. Discussion of the problem with the patient and his wife revealed that the impotency did not worry her, that she had never expected much in the way of sexual relations when she married the patient, and that she would gladly give up her job to please him.

EPILOGUE

To some, the approaches advocated herein may seem superficial. We would like to remind these believers "in depth" of the realities of 2,600 new patients a year in a general medical clinic and in a busy practitioner's office. Furthermore, we would like to say a few things in explanation.

Much of our present-day medical and paramedical ethos conceives of unusual personality patterns as "sick." Thus labels like masochistic or obsessive-compulsive become equivalent to entities like poliomyelitis or adenocarcinoma. This kind of thinking implies that everyone should have a "normal" personality pattern and that the possession of such a pattern will preclude emotional illness. Therapeutic efforts, if any, are bent toward altering the patient's personality toward this idealized norm. Such alterations, however, are not only difficult to accomplish but generally impractical. Perhaps this is a good thing because a world of such uniformity would be dreadfully dull. Furthermore, the assumption that a person's basic personality must change before he can be helped and that that change can occur only with intensive and prolonged recall of childhood experiences allows both patient and physician to do nothing about the problems at hand.

Most of psychiatry and psychology is concerned with the conceptualized "why" of personality patterns — why is this person a masochist, why that one an obsessive-compulsive, and so forth? In this book, we have attempted to teach recognition of the patient's personality pattern, acceptance of the person for what he is, formulation of a plan of management for his current problems, and noninterference with this plan by the emotions engendered in the physician by the patient. There is, for example, a considerable difference between telling the scrubwoman married to a sadistic, alcoholic husband: "There is no medical cure for you, you can live with him or leave him, but getting 'sick' is no solution" and the approach which tells the patient she is a masochist because of early childhood experiences, the effects of which must be eliminated before she can change.

Not only is the first approach more practical in a

busy clinic or office but, in addition, it offers much
more than simply recognizing that we cannot promise
that medical science, through some pill, nostrum, or
conceptualization will cure this particular illness or
all the illness in the world. A clear definition of what
medical science can or cannot do and what the patient's own responsibility is has lowered significantly
the number of chronically returning "thick-chart" patients. The approach which we advocate is not one of
shrugging off medical responsibilities and rejecting
the troubled patient. It involves much in the way of
support, understanding, tolerance, elaboration of
alternatives, and encouragement of independent de-
cision-making.

Basic to this view is our respect for free will. By
contrast, most of medical science today seems to favor
determinism and linear causality. Of course, for the
purpose of arriving at useful abstractions, it is easier
for science to order events in a causal chain and to
view a person and his behavior as the consequence
thereof. The causes of behavior are then reified: Some
one thing — a poor home environment, a conflict, a
weak super-ego — causes the patient (determines
him) to act in a certain manner. This absolution
from personal responsibility can have serious consequences for society. On the other hand, the advoca-
tion of free will, of personal choice, of decision, favors

self-determination, individuality, and responsibility. No longer is the physician the possessor of the magic that will find *it*, the cause, and exorcise it from the patient. No longer can the patient (and the physician) evade necessary decisions, while pleading lack of funds, time, or facilities to seek out the presumed, conceptualized, approximate causes of the disturbance. It must be realized too that making no decision is a decision in itself and the patient may decide then to live with the problem.

Nevertheless, even as we write this, we are conscious that, in this epilogue, we are dealing with words, with intellectual concepts, rather than people. As is commonly said, "The map is not the territory," or, "There are no diseases, there are only sick people." We have no desire to occupy ourselves in intellectual discussions at the expense of involvement with the realities of patients' existences. Only the results of these methods with the patients in the physician's office will decide the issues.